The Dieter's Guide to Success

Audrey Eyton, former beauty editor of *Woman*, was the founder-editor of *Slimming* magazine. She continues to be editorial director of this highly successful publication which now owns a nationwide chain of slimming clubs and a health farm, Ragdale Hall. Audrey Eyton's many years of specialization in the problems of weight control have earned her the reputation of being Britain's most informed writer on the subject.

Henry Jordan, Clinical Associate Professor of Psychiatry at the School of Medicine, University of Pennsylvania, is one of America's leading psychiatrists in the field of weight control. He graduated from Harvard College and from the University of Pennsylvania. In 1976 Dr Jordan founded the Institute for Behavioral Education to conduct research and to offer clinical treatment for the obese.

The Dieter's Guide to Success

100 ways to beat temptation and get slim

Audrey Eyton and Dr Henry Jordan

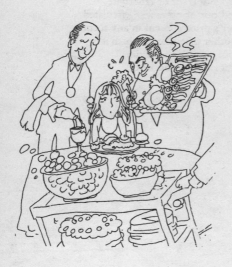

FONTANA PAPERBACKS

First published by Fontana Paperbacks 1981

Made and printed in Great Britain by
William Collins Sons & Co. Ltd, Glasgow

Contents

6 *Contents*

Introduction

You don't intend to eat, you are determined *not* to eat. YOU EAT! Why?

There can be at least a hundred different reasons why people trying to control or reduce their body weight succumb to overeating or diet breaking. The world around us is a minefield of appetite-triggering temptations. You will be able to step through it much more safely after reading this book.

If we are unaware of the dangers, our appetites can be triggered off by something as slight as a chance comment from a friend, or our dieting efforts can be sabotaged by carefully calculated commercial interests. Considering all the hazards, it isn't at all surprising that so many people fail to control their weight – more of a miracle that some *do* succeed in weight-loss programmes.

You will take a big stride forward to success just by becoming *aware* of all the eating temptations around you. In this book we tell you the most effective ways to defuse each temptation, but awareness is the main key to success. It's the unexpected or unrecognized temptation that is most likely to throw you. That was the one which broke your willpower in the past!

Don't worry if some of the advice in this book seems to conflict with established ideas on weight control. It does indeed – and very deliberately! If you always thought, for instance, that you *must* start the day with a good breakfast, you may be surprised to find yourself being told not to eat this meal unless you genuinely feel hungry first thing in the morning. If the need for three 'proper' meals each day has been instilled into you, you may even be shocked to be told that if all you are really yearning for at lunch time is a slice of fruit pie, all you need eat is that slice of fruit pie.

Man cannot live on fruit pie alone. A healthy diet needs to consist of varied foods. But much of the nutritional advice still in circulation emanated from the days when malnutrition was a prevalent problem of the Western world. Today nutritional deficiencies are rare in our affluent society and the major nutritional problem is 'overnutrition'. Most of us are getting all the minerals, vitamins and protein that we need, and even more than we need, and an excess doesn't do us any more good than just enough.

Certainly it is unnecessary to eat three meals a day in order to stay healthy. The three-meal pattern is simply a social convention. In the days when malnutrition was a problem in this country it also seemed a good idea to recommend this regular eating pattern as a precaution against deficiencies. These days, however, much of the advice aimed at preventing these problems of the past is inadvertently encouraging calorie excesses.

People remain convinced that they must eat those three 'proper' meals daily, so they eat them. But at the same time they are using up less calories, in this mechanized age, and being tempted, by all the situations you will read about, to consume extra calories in drinks and snacks. The result is the excess calories which lead to excess weight.

The solutions lie both in reducing habit-based eating and moderating the impulsive eating which is triggered off by the temptations dealt with in this book.

Another reason why the advice you will read may conflict with advice you have been given in the past is that so much scientific research into obesity has been based on experiments with rats. Rats are different from people! Rats don't have to contend with television advertisements for chocolate-coated munchy bars, or the siren call of the office tea trolley – things which can so easily make your mind want to carry on eating when your stomach is quite satisfied.

Two factors can trigger off the urge to eat. One of these is hunger, which depends on the state of fullness of the stomach. The other factor is 'appetite', which has little to do with the stomach. Appetite is a desire to eat triggered off by the sight, smell or anticipated taste of a particular food. If, after a reasonably substantial lunch, you find that by mid-afternoon you are very tempted to eat a slice of cake because someone happens to offer you a slice of your favourite cake, you are responding to appetite, not hunger.

Old-style diet advice was geared very much to protecting people from hunger. Modern experts like psychiatrist Dr Henry Jordan are more and more convinced that appetite is the major factor in causing people to consume excess calories.

Eating is a necessary and a pleasurable occupation and this book is designed to protect you only from eating the calories you didn't intend to eat at the times when you didn't intend to eat them. It is the perfect companion book to any diet. Diets tell only half the story: they tell you what to eat and what *not* to eat – but never tell you *how* not to eat it! Little wonder that so many diets fail by neglecting this essential, psychological half of the story. After reading this book you will be armed to deal with those eating temptations of the future which floored your weight-control efforts in the past. This time you will really discover 'what went wrong before' and learn how to cope with the unknown appetite triggers which you probably simply interpreted as lack-of-willpower.

Final word: we don't expect you to resist a hundred temptations one hundred per cent of the time. But once you have recognized the temptations, many will automatically cancel themselves out; others you will learn how to cope with. By curing your vulnerability to unexpected temptations you will be well on your way to achieving that elusive goal of permanent weight control – at last.

Aggravations

Not very long ago an overweight patient who had embarked, with great determination, on a weight-reduction programme, reported in for her first week's progress check. She was shame-faced, disappointed, and to come and explain her failure had probably taken a good deal of effort.

No, she hadn't succeeded in keeping to the calorie goals she had set herself, she hadn't lost any weight. She'd set off well enough, splendidly in fact. For the first two days she had really done well in putting into practice the new eating-control methods she was starting to learn. But then the *darndest* thing happened. . . .

Coming home after a very pleasant day out with a friend, she discovered that something had gone wrong with the washing machine which she had switched on before she left home. In fact, something had gone *very* wrong. The kitchen floor was flooded, so were the mats and the carpet in the hall. She was furious. The soggy, half-washed clothes would have to be fished out of the machine. The floor would have to be mopped and the carpets dried, the washing-machine company would have to be called in, and she wasn't quite sure where she had listed their phone number. . . .

Peeling off her shoes and stockings, she paddled through the kitchen and put on the kettle. Then she paddled to the pantry and got out a packet of chocolate digestive biscuits. Before she had finished munching and fuming, about three-quarters of the packet of biscuits had gone, and after that there didn't seem to be much point counting her calories for the rest of the day, or week!

The link between mechanical failure and excessive calorie intake would seem an obscure one. Yet haven't you found yourself turning to food during moments of major or minor aggravation like this? The car won't start, the TV breaks down, the plumber who had promised to turn up just doesn't turn up . . . and, without really realizing why, you find yourself eating.

The petty annoyances of life can provide people with a considerable temptation to turn to extra snacks, and, like the other temptations you will read about in this book, there is a perfectly logical reason for this seemingly illogical link between a broken washing machine and three-quarters of a packet of chocolate digestive biscuits.

Food can be a marvellous reliever of aggravation and frustration. During early childhood we were often taught by parents that when things went wrong an ice-cream cone or a lollypop would make us feel much better. These associations continue all our lives. Because in the past we have experienced relief by eating food, we tend to turn to it now as almost an automatic reflex action.

Eating also gives us an excuse to take a break from the aggravation, and delays the effort that is usually going to be involved in rectifying the problem. You see, eating provides a good excuse to delay doing things – the things we don't want to have to do – at certain times.

Oddly enough, people rarely allow themselves to say, 'That was an infuriating thing to happen – but I'm going to take ten minutes before doing something about it,' *unless* they have a specific reason for taking a break, like having a cup of coffee and a snack. That is acceptable to them, so that is what they do.

So when aggravations arise in your life – and they will! – what can you do to resist the temptation to turn to extra snacks?

Well, if you hate the thought of coping with the problem, consider first whether there is any alternative way of taking a break and easing the frustration and aggravation before you tackle it. Possibly a phone call to a friend would prove therapeutic because it would allow you, during the conversation, to mention that the ! ! ! washing machine just overflowed; and voicing a frustration helps to relieve it.

Another possible solution to this temptation – it may not knock it out completely, but often it cuts it down – is to set up a policy that when something aggravating happens you will wait at least ten minutes before turning to food. During that ten minutes you can make a very deliberate decision about whether to eat and what to eat. We find that when delays like this are put into aggravation-response eating quite often people will decide that no, they really don't need food. If they do decide to go ahead and eat they will do it in a much more controlled way. Usually they will decide that what they need is just one small portion of food. They are much less likely to go into the kitchen in a frenzy, opening cupboards and picking up anything available, in a strong emotional response to aggravation.

When aggravations arise, try to do something other than eating to relieve your feelings. And if you can't resist eating, at least delay eating until your feelings are under control.

Bargain eating

One of the most universally popular indoor sports is a game called Beat the Restaurant. Most of us are eager contestants. The aim of the game, having committed yourself to paying a set price for a restaurant meal, is to eat anything and everything available in order to win the satisfaction of having got 'good value'.

You win if you eat *everything*. Even if you don't like soup you must eat the soup if it is included in the price.

The restaurant wins if you skip a course or even refuse a bread roll. You are left with the uncomfortable feeling that you haven't got full value for money, and that the restaurant has made more profit out of you than it really ought.

However, you are unlikely to lose because another key rule of this game is that the waiters and waitresses, plus your eating companions, are all on your side. Should you impulsively decide to miss a course, or refuse the baked potato because you don't really want it, someone can always be relied upon to remind you: 'It's all included in the price, you know. . . .' Then you find yourself hesitating and changing your mind: 'Oh, all right, perhaps I will. . . .'

The competitive spirit reaches its peak in the help-yourself restaurants – where, for a set sum, you are allowed to pile your plate as high as you like. Here's where the sporting person really scents a challenge. In fact these restaurants were set up to capitalize on that universal urge to feel that we are 'eating a bargain'!

Never underestimate that powerful urge to eat all the food you have paid for. It is a major eating temptation that accounts for many unnecessary calories being consumed. Even the most careless spenders in other directions tend to suffer from an instinctive frugal urge in this direction.

Since we are all tempted to eat all the food we have paid for, the safest bet, generally, is to choose a restaurant where you only pay for the food you really want to eat. Inclusive three-course meals and help-yourself counters tempt us into the money trap.

On an *à la carte* menu the money factor aids self control. The more food you order, the more you have to pay. And restaurants which supply only an *à la carte* menu are usually more expensive. In choosing your restaurant, consider how much money you have to spend and whether you could get one really delicious course at a good restaurant in place of a three-course meal at a cheaper one. Aim at getting value in quality, rather than quantity of food.

Generally you are much less likely to fall into the money trap if you recognize that you are getting value in service as well as food in a restaurant. Remind yourself that you don't have to shop for the meal or prepare it or serve it or do the washing up afterwards. Add this service value into your sums when you tot up what you are paying for your food.

Big packs

Are you strong-willed, *really* strong-willed? Then try to stop before you've finished off that bar of chocolate, or to leave that packet of potato crisps or peanuts still part full.

Few people have that degree of willpower, and the compelling urge to finish off that pack of snackable food is one of the strongest eating temptations. With these foods we have deeply conditioned ourselves to use only the sight of an empty pack as a stop mechanism. Only when we see it empty do we feel satisfied.

There are commendable exceptions to this urge-to-finish-off-the-unit rule. The late Bing Crosby was one. 'He was the only man I knew,' remarked his widow, Cathy, 'who had sufficient self-discipline to eat only half a biscuit!'

But, unless your willpower puts you in the superstar bracket, this temptation can be so strong that it is much wiser to pander to it than fight it.

Accept that the size of the packet or bar you buy dictates the quantity you will eat. So, if you buy a small pack you will naturally consume less calories than if you bought a big one.

Use self-control at purchase point, which is the easiest time.

Buy small!

Blue moods

Blue moods – which even the cheeriest among us suffer from time to time – can be bad news in food control.

Severe depression sometimes leads to loss of appetite, but, more often, depressed moods tempt us to turn to food.

Depressed people tend to turn to food for comfort because the blue mood tends to negate most alternatives. When we are in these moods we usually withdraw from other people, and lack the energy and desire to get ourselves involved in activities which could turn out to be pleasurable. Apathy takes over, and food is the only comfort which seems available. But, unfortunately for the overweight person, this 'comfort eating' usually intensifies the degree of depression.

To resist this temptation it is necessary to lift the mood. And that means changing those blue thoughts – thoughts that we aren't very adequate or capable of solving our problems and that nothing good is going to happen to solve them for us – which are usually an integral part of depression.

Many psychiatrists are convinced that the best way for a person to alleviate a depressed mood is to become involved in any kind of task which they can successfully complete. Even severely depressed people respond well to simple tasks which they have been given as part of their therapy.

Feeling blue? Then *do* something. Oddly enough, you will usually find it easier to persuade yourself to do something not particularly pleasant, like a long-put-off household task, than something designed only to give pleasure. A certain degree of masochism is often associated with a depressed mood; there is almost an urge to want to wallow in misery. In this kind of mood you are unlikely to persuade yourself to do something enjoyable, because you won't believe that you would enjoy it! You will often find yourself more responsive to the idea: 'Might as well have a *thoroughly* miserable time, as I'm feeling miserable already. . . .'

Having accomplished any small task – washing the car, tidying a cupboard – you are likely to start experiencing a definite lift in mood. Even a minor accomplishment starts to counteract the basic feeling of helplessness and inadequacy. The important thing is to be able to tell yourself: 'I have done something constructive.' In many cases this can generate enough energy to make you want to go on and do something else. And the more you accomplish, the more your mood is likely to change.

We remember one patient, several years ago, who had obviously worked this out for herself. An unmarried mother, she often had to spend evenings alone at home, and one of the reasons for her weight problem was the extra eating that took place during these lonely and often depressing evenings. Resolved to shed weight, she hit on the idea of what she came to describe as her 'thoroughly nasty nights', during which nothing that needed washing remained unwashed, or unmended, and aunts who had been owed letters for years were at last rewarded.

Her obvious high spirits after these episodes, and her success in eventually shedding all her surplus weight, testified to the effectiveness of her 'if I'm going to be miserable I might as well do something useful' attitude.

For the overweight person, the great fringe benefit of doing something practical during a blue mood is that, at least while you are doing it, you are less likely to succumb to the temptation to eat. Nothing raises the dieter's spirits more than success in resisting extra food. You start to feel a little bit pleased with yourself for doing something useful, then even *more* pleased with yourself for keeping to your diet, and it is almost impossible to feel depressed when you are feeling pleased with yourself.

Boredom

Boredom is without doubt the mood which most tempts you to eat. You are even more likely to snack if you are bored than you are if you are depressed – although the two moods are often linked.

If a lifestyle survey were taken on people who find it easy to control their weight, and on those who find it very difficult, we strongly suspect that the former would turn out to be people who are always busy and mentally involved with work and activities.

When they embark on a weight-loss campaign most people give considerable thought to what they will eat, and what they won't eat. Few people give any thought to what they will *do*. Yet this factor can be absolutely crucial in deciding whether that campaign will succeed or not.

Our patients are strongly encouraged to take up new activities as part of their slimming programme. They are even asked to report on progress in these directions at weekly consultations. We find, in studying the lifestyles of overweight people, that very often all their activity is centred around the family and that they aren't actually involved in anything which is designed to give them pleasure and interest as individuals.

You will probably have to overcome considerable apathy and habitual resistance before you can contemplate what would get you out of the house more, or occupy and interest you when you have to stay at home. You will be tempted to tell yourself: 'Well, I shall start doing more once I reach my goal weight!'

This is a dangerous attitude. If you experience frequent periods of boredom in your life you are very unlikely to keep to your diet and reach your target weight.

So make definite plans to beat boredom – the most snack-inducing mood – as an integral part of your slimming campaign.

Bread rolls

You do not go to a restaurant to eat bread rolls and butter. You could stay at home and eat bread and butter! Yet the procedure of most restaurants provides a very strong temptation to eat these foods in the form of rather unnecessary calories – and calories which are surplus to the meal.

In almost any restaurant, the custom is for the waiter to place the rolls and butter on the table as soon as you sit down. Then he may go away for a little while before he takes the order. Then maybe there is a gap of ten or fifteen minutes before the first course arrives. During all this period you are sitting, feeling rather hungry, with bread in front of you. So you find yourself starting to nibble it, probably with quite a lavish amount of butter which supplies more calories than the bread.

What can you do to avoid this situation? The perfect solution to the problem is to ask the waiter not to place the bread on the table. If the restaurant follows the procedure of just placing one roll on each person's plate, it is easy enough to say 'No thank you' when he is about to give you yours. It is rather more difficult if a basket of rolls is placed on the table, because this means refusing on behalf of everyone else.

So the next step, if the rolls do end up on the table, is to move them away from you. Pass the basket to somebody else and let the rolls and the temptation they provide sit in front of somebody else, so that at least, if you are going to have one, you have to go to the trouble of asking for the basket to be passed to you.

To lessen the temptation to eat bread while you are awaiting your meal it is a very good idea to have a drink, which helps while away the time. You could ask for a glass of water or a low-calorie beverage; better still, ask for a cup of coffee to be served immediately, before the meal. Although the usual custom is for coffee to be served at the end of the meal, few restaurants will refuse this reasonable request. Remember, in a restaurant you are paying for service as well as food. Most people get over-concerned with getting full value from food – too little concerned with getting full value from the service.

Breakfast ('I *always* eat it!')

Many people who don't feel hungry at the start of the day always eat breakfast because . . . well, because they *always* eat breakfast! Habit is a key factor in many eating temptations. Habits feature prominently in dictating all our actions at the start of the day.

Nearly everything we do, from climbing out of bed always from the same side, to cleaning our teeth always before or always after washing, to the order in which we put on our clothes, follows an intriguingly set and habitual pattern during the first waking hour.

Breakfast is the most habitual meal of the day in content. People who would protest if served the same lunch on two consecutive days will happily eat two slices of buttered toast and marmalade for breakfast, day after day after day.

People who don't eat breakfast tend *never* to eat breakfast on a normal working day.

People who eat breakfast *always* eat breakfast. When real hunger is absent, this is often why they are eating breakfast – because it has become a set part of their early-morning habitual routine. That routine can strongly tempt us either to eat or not to eat. To switch from one to the other demands deliberate effort at first –but it may pay off. You may discover, as the new habit becomes entrenched, that you have been eating breakfast entirely out of habit – not hunger.

Breakfast ('You *ought* to eat it!')

Some people eat breakfast because they feel hungry early in the morning.

Many other people don't feel hungry, but eat break-fast because they feel they really 'ought' to eat it. Thus they succumb to the temptation to consume calories at the time of day when they could most easily avoid food altogether.

Not hungry? Surely, after the long fast of the night . . . ? Yes, it does seem illogical. But after studying hundreds of case histories, in which overweight people recorded their feelings of hunger throughout the day, we find that the early morning is the time when most people feel least hungry. What is more, many people find that if they skip breakfast they don't feel hungry during the morning, while if they eat breakfast they actually feel hungrier during the morning.

Recent scientific research suggests an explanation for these strange findings. It seems probable that after the stomach has been emptied during the night the body starts its own fat-burning mechanism. As part of this process, chemical substances are produced, which are now thought to have an appetite-suppressing side-effect.

This also helps to explain some other well-known

appetite-loss phenomena – why people who starve for lengthy periods usually lose their appetites, and why people who delay meals often find that they have 'passed the stage of wanting it'.

But if you have been brought up to believe that you 'ought' to eat breakfast, the chances are that you've never really noticed that you aren't hungry at breakfast time. Like a patient of ours who enrolled for a course of early-morning weight-control sessions and only realized, after a number of weeks, that in order to keep her early appointment on this particular day she had been skipping her usual breakfast without feeling any ill effects, and without experiencing any greater hunger during the morning or at lunch time. From then on she labelled breakfast as unnecessary calories, and cut it out completely.

As well as the many people who eat breakfast because 'they feel they ought to', there are many more who eat it because someone else feels they ought to, fond mothers and wives in particular. We had one patient whose thirty-pound-surplus-weight problem was caused entirely by breakfast. Throughout his adult life he had been in the habit of having nothing but coffee in the morning. Then he divorced and remarried, choosing for his second wife a very devoted lady who took care of his socks and shirts and home with loving care, and insisted on cooking him 'the good breakfast he needed' on which to start the working day.

By eating his usual lunch and dinner and drinking his usual drinks over the years, our patient had obviously been consuming just enough to keep his weight steady. By adding breakfast to his calorie total he now started consuming just too much. And so his weight gradually but steadily rose. . . .

'Stop eating breakfast,' was our advice on locating the cause of the problem.

'But my wife thinks I ought to eat breakfast, isn't she right . . .?'

'Well, did you suffer any ill effects *before,* during all those years when you didn't eat breakfast?'

Putting it to a personal test is probably the best answer to the common folklore, assisted by a somewhat debatable survey of a few years ago, which has put into people's minds the idea that 'you ought to eat breakfast'. Millions of people don't eat breakfast, and suffer no ill effects. Those who are used to breakfast may suffer from some hunger or lack of concentration during the morning when they break the habit, but these feelings are unlikely to persist.

Certainly no informed medical expert would suggest that skipping breakfast could have any ill effects on the health of the normal, adult person.

This shouldn't imply that no one ought to eat breakfast. Appetite and hunger patterns vary, and for some people this is a hungry time of the day. But don't be tempted to eat breakfast just because you feel you 'ought to', because many people eat unnecessary calories this way.

Business lunches

Whisper it quietly – nobody really likes to admit to this – but one of the main temptations presented by a business lunch is the thought that you can indulge in a high quality meal for free. Usually your company or his company is paying the bill. Free food is a great appetite stimulant.

Another harder-to-tackle appetite stimulant is the sight of all those people around you eating all that lovely food. You could, of course, choose only low-calorie dishes like grilled fish. But if richer dishes always prove very tempting in these situations the best solution is to eat extremely sparingly during the remainder of the day to allow for lunch-time indulgences.

Even when you order rich dishes at that hungry moment before the meal, you can often recoup the situation by taking a split second, during the course of the meal, to ask yourself: 'Do I really need to continue to eat this food?' A good deal of mindless eating goes on at business lunches. Once absorbed in conversation you may well find that you are continuing to put food in your mouth simply because it is there before you. You may find it easy to put down your knife and fork part way through a course. Usually no one else will notice, and in these weight-conscious days restrained eating tends to create a good rather than a poor impression.

The alcoholic calories tend to be a little more difficult to handle, particularly if you are a host hoping that a few drinks will put your guest in a relaxed and agreeable frame of mind. Obviously, if you don't drink, your guest will feel restrained in this direction.

One businessman we know found a well-planned solution to this problem. Like most businessmen who entertain frequently, he tended to use the same small group of convenient restaurants where he was a well-known figure. Here it was easy enough for him to arrange with the waiters that whenever he ordered a martini for himself he should simply be served a martini-glass of water.

A compromise solution is to drink only the drinks which will be noticed, which are those ordered before the meal. Few people are aware of how much wine anyone has consumed during the course of a meal. Usually the waiter refills the glasses without anyone noticing. By keeping your glass full you can avoid the refills without having to refuse them. Keep a glass of water by your wine-glass and nobody will notice which one you sip.

Business lunches are tempting occasions, but there are many ways to cut down their calorie content, and in no way need they provide an insuperable obstacle to controlling weight.

Cafeteria coffee traps

Every time you go into a self-service cafeteria 'just for a coffee', count on the following chain of events:

1. You will pick up your tray.
2. You will discover that the coffee is being dispensed right at the far end of the counter, and between you and it lies a long array of food.
3. There is a line of people in front of you, so it is impossible to dash past the food.
4. As you stand nose-to-slice with eye-level food displays you will discover, to your surprise, that, yes, you are a little peckish, and minute by minute even that rather yellowed pastry will grow in jammy charm.
5. You will be tempted. . . .

Don't go into a cafeteria 'just for a coffee' unless you are aware that you are stepping into a situation deliberately designed to tempt you to eat – and are strong enough to walk the gauntlet with eyes averted!

Cakes (large)

A large cake, one which you buy or bake for the family, can provide you with a considerable eating temptation for several days.

It's fairly safe before you cut it. You're hardly going to present it at the table in a form which provides indisputable evidence against you. A large chunk, already cut out, reveals that 'you couldn't wait', and exactly how much you ate. Few people who are sensitive about their weight are going to risk the jokes that might ensue!

But, once that cake is cut it becomes a ticking time-bomb. The large portion left offers a constant temptation to slice off a little bit more, and a little bit more . . . and no one will know how much you ate. Also the cut face of a cake is usually even more tempting to the appetite than the top of an uncut cake.

You'll tell yourself that you'll just cut off a mere 'shaving' – maybe even just a handful of crumbs. Then, an hour later, maybe just another tiny, tiny taste. . . .

For this reason, it's a pretty unwise idea to buy or bake a large cake for the family. If you're baking, it's much easier to bake two smaller cakes. If you have a freezer, freeze one of them so that it's safe from instant-nibbling temptation. You can also consider freezing the leftover half of a cake.

Another solution – if you have just enough of the cake left for one more family serving – would be to slice it (one slice each), immediately foil-wrap to store, and serve on the table in slices. To combat your nibbling temptations you have the thought of the nasty scenes that will ensue if there isn't one slice left for everybody!

Cakes (small) and pastries

If you are tempted to have a small cake or pastry, buy one – *only* one! This is the only way to ensure that you eat just one.

Don't feel obliged to buy cakes in popular units like 'half a dozen'. If you are buying for the family, buy one for each member of the family, five (not six!) cakes for a family of five. That odd leftover cake is the one that will most tempt you – usually it 'disappears' before the family even sets eyes on it.

Self-control takes only a few seconds in the cake shop but if you buy surplus cakes it takes hours of self-control to avoid eating them.

Cheesecake

For many people, cheesecake presents an instant combination of a multitude of charms.

Cheesecake is a particularly exciting combination of varied food textures (often both smooth and crunchy) and varied food tastes (both sharp and sweet). Kept in the kitchen it becomes an instantly available source of what might be described as 'taste thrills' — the kind of eating sensations we are seeking when we tire of bland-tasting diet foods.

Nothing else tastes quite like cheesecake. So if you are tempted to eat it, no other food will curb the craving. And it is particularly difficult to stop eating cheesecake once you have started, because variety stimulates the appetite and here you get a whole variety of tastes and textures all in one food. It is a food which particularly lends itself to the repeated 'I'll just have one more spoonful' trap.

To think you can buy a whole cheesecake, then only eat one slice, is often a big mistake. If you must (and we'd rather you didn't!), at least ensure that there is no more cheesecake than the family can demolish at the next meal, because leftover pieces of cheesecake are a near-irresistible temptation to many people. Even if you have learned the art of throwing leftovers away, anticipate special difficulties here. Some foods, we find, are more difficult to throw away than others. Cheesecake is one of the most difficult.

By far the best way to prevent cheesecake binges is to restrict cheesecake eating to restaurants, where you will be served a single portion only. If a passing glimpse of cheesecake causes a craving, try to satisfy it in a one-slice-only situation, either by eating it in a café with a coffee, or buying from a shop which sells individual slices.

For many people this is the kind of food which is only

on the mind if it is also in the kitchen. Keeping it out of the kitchen is the best way to keep it out of the mind.

Chocolate

There seems to be some special magical quality in the taste and texture of chocolate which makes it the subject of so many strong cravings.

Kept in the house it provides a totally irresistible temptation to many people at many times. To keep it out of the house you need to persuade other members of the family not to bring it in! No point in urging them to 'hide it away'; you will sense its presence, seek it out like a cigaretteless nicotine addict searching pockets for stubs, if you suffer strong chocolate cravings.

Chocolate cravings know no honesty. We've known otherwise impeccable mothers stoop to stealing their own children's chocolate bars, and recall one upright citizen confessing that she was 'almost prepared to smash a shop-window' to obtain a bar of chocolate one evening. We know the feeling!

Most people seem to experience chocolate cravings – but with a degree of frequency varying from almost every day to only once or twice a year. Unfortunately, the more frequently you eat it the more often you start to crave it! So the less-strong cravings need to be resisted to cut down frequency. This is best achieved by ensuring that chocolate isn't instantly available in the home, and by trying at least to delay buying chocolate by getting involved in other things which may distract your mind.

If a craving persists, despite a reasonable amount of delay and distraction, it is better to satisfy it with a small quantity rather than risk it building up into a binge. Use your control at purchase point: buy only one small bar.

Be assertive in asking friends and relatives not to buy

you chocolate gifts. Not only will you polish off the chocolate given – you will be more inclined to buy yourself more chocolate when that is finished. Don't buy other people chocolate, either – you know they'll offer you some!

People have found many different ways to decrease their chocolate cravings, and it pays to be experimental. One woman we know decided to eat only the most expensive chocolates with fillings made from real fruits, and was gratified to find that lesser products began to taste unpleasantly synthetic. By becoming a chocolate gourmet she cost-limited chocolate eating to an occasional treat and eliminated the temptation of everyday products. A model girl we know discovered that she could satisfy her cravings with one bite – as long as she immediately threw the rest of the bar into the dustbin. A hairdresser experimented with sweets to find 'the next best substitute' and discovered that he could resist chocolate as long as he ate peppermints. Then he gradually weaned himself off peppermints. . . .

Don't rely on willpower alone to increase your resistance to this temptation. Tackle the problem with imagination and ingenuity to find your own best solution.

Cleaning your plate

Learning to control your weight is probably going to mean defying your mother. This may take a little courage and persistence, even if you are now sixty-two!

Good little boys and girls always clean their plates. This was imprinted in your mind, probably even before you could speak, as your mother carefully scraped out that bowl of soggy cereal and shoved the last teaspoon between your pursed and petulant lips.

This is a tough one to tackle.

You're going to have to tackle it sooner or later, because

it's the bad boys and girls who defied their mothers who usually become thin adults. Look around in any restaurant and you will see that it is usually the slim people who have left some of their food, while all the overweight people have cleared their plates.

This deeply imprinted maternal lesson provides you with a constant temptation to eat more than you really need, and even more than you really want. It negates all your natural STOP mechanisms. You become programmed to stop eating only at one signal – the sight of an empty plate. You will eat all that is placed before you, however much that may be.

It takes very deliberate practice and awareness to change a lifelong habit. Practise leaving at least a little food on your plate at every meal. Do this deliberately. At first you won't want to do it – but do it.

Then start asking yourself, 'Have I had enough, do I really need any more?' at some stage during each meal. Eventually you will find that you really have had enough and don't feel the need to clean your plate. Still later you will discover that you simply *can't* clean your plate when someone has served you with an overlarge portion.

It all takes time and practice but this is worthwhile because re-acquiring natural STOP mechanisms in eating is a major factor in becoming able to control your weight.

Clocks

Your mind is absorbed in one of the tasks of the morning. Suddenly, out of the corner of your eye, you catch sight of the clock. Goodness, it is one o'clock – it is lunch time – you are hungry! Those thoughts follow each other in quick succession. Had you not noticed the time you may well have carried on working without giving a thought to food. The clock has tempted you to eat.

One of the major differences in behaviour we have found between overweight and effortlessly slim people is that slim people are much less likely to be bullied into eating by the clock. When the clock indicates a mealtime the slim person is more able to say, 'So what!' and decide to delay a meal. And delayed meals are often missed altogether.

In contrast, our eating records show that overweight people almost universally show a faithful devotion to eating their main meals at almost precisely the same time of day, each day. Often they will go to great trouble to avoid delaying meals. We remember one patient who actually brought a packed lunch in her car when she started attending weight-control sessions, just in case her lengthy drive home delayed her lunch.

People who are not bullied by the clock gain a natural advantage in calorie control by taking effortless advantage of those situations, such as an extra-busy schedule, which tempt us *not* to eat. This is one of the reasons why they do not have weight problems.

If your appetite is dominated by the clock, work at defeating this bully. Start looking for natural opportunities to delay and skip meals – even create some by getting involved in tasks, journeys and outings which will keep you involved at times when you would normally be eating.

At first you may find this a little uncomfortable. The clock actually has the power to summon up hunger pangs – often you only start to feel them when you notice the time! But people who often delay and miss meals usually acquire the capability of going for lengthy periods without food, without experiencing physical discomfort. This is a useful capability to acquire.

Regular meals, at the same time of day each day, are a social habit rather than a health requirement for the adult person in normal health.

Time is certainly against you in your weight-control efforts as long as you allow that clock to dictate your meals.

Clothes kept 'just in case'

You are progressing well on your diet, you are shedding weight, you are actually discovering – oh joy of joys! – that some of your clothes are becoming too big and baggy. So what do you do with them?

What many people do is to keep their too-big clothes 'just in case'!

Not a good idea. By keeping those clothes, you are telling yourself: 'I'm going to fail.' This can be a self-fulfilling prophecy. You will be more tempted to weaken during a difficult period if you haven't burned your bridges (or clothes!) behind you.

On the other hand, it is probably asking a little too much of human courage and confidence to ask you to throw out all your 'fat' clothes as soon as you start to get slimmer. The best compromise solution is to throw or give away items of clothing, one piece at a time, as your weight loss progresses. You make a decision, for instance, to get rid of one item of overlarge clothing as you shed each seven, eight or nine pounds.

Cocktail parties

To emerge with self-control intact from all the calorie temptations of a cocktail party depends on a very definite plan of campaign, rather than an optimistic spirit.

How many alcoholic drinks are you going to allow yourself?

How many hors d'oeuvres are you going to eat?

How long are you going to stay?

If you make those three decisions in advance, you arrive well armed to moderate your eating and drinking. If you don't feel that you can afford to spend any calories at all, you would probably be better staying at home.

An advance decision on the quantity of food and drink allows you to work out the least sacrificial way of keeping to that quantity. If you decide to have three alcoholic drinks, and plan to stay for about one and a half hours, you have the option of starting on low-calorie soft drinks and switching to alcohol later, or perhaps alternating each alcoholic drink with a low-calorie drink.

Many of the alcoholic calories consumed at cocktail parties slip down without being noticed. This is because people stand with glasses in their hands. Then they become involved in animated conversation. During the conversation the glass repeatedly raises itself to their lips. Only when the glass becomes surprisingly empty does the glass-holder start to become aware of what it has been up to.

To protect yourself against the independent movement of your glass, do not hold it while you are involved in a conversation. Place it on some table or shelf. This also protects you from your host when he comes round to refill your glass. You can point in some vaguely indeterminate direction and assure him: 'It's over there and still full, thanks — I'll let you know when I'm ready!'

Hands can move independently, too, so don't stand in arm's reach of the peanuts.

Cocktail party food has an unpredictable quality. There's a great temptation to help yourself to the first hors d'oeuvres offered around, because you don't know what you will be offered next, or even when it will be offered. 'Better help myself now while I have the chance,' is a natural reaction. Often, hot even–more–succulent goodies arrive after you've already indulged in a generous quantity of cold snacks. A decision to allow yourself only a set number of snacks makes you more inclined to resist the first offerings until you see what else is available.

Usually no one else is aware of what you eat and drink at a cocktail party, and a few little white lies – 'No thanks, I've had three of those already and they're delicious' – can best protect you from being pressed to eat food which you are trying to resist. The important thing is to remain aware of it yourself by eating and drinking according to plan, not according to the number of times you are offered food and drink.

Coffee break

In most offices, every day and usually at the same time of day, around comes the snack trolley – loaded with temptations. Usually it carries the same foods, often some very tasty and tempting pastry products.

Usually everyone partakes, whether they are hungry or not, because it is also a signal that you can take a little break from your work. Taking some food at coffee break is a socially acceptable excuse for not working for a little while. Eating is often used as an excuse for not doing other things.

One has to accept that this is going to be a very tempting event. There's the presence of food, the need to take a little break from work, the fact that everyone else is going to patronize the snack trolley and that while they do a certain amount of pleasant socialization usually goes on.

You have to start by asking yourself how important the food itself really is to you, compared to the other pleasant factors involved. If the food isn't really all that important, then you can take the break and enjoy the socialization without having to eat the pastry. Just have the tea or coffee.

If the food itself really is going to tempt you, then you can get right away from it by using another reason for taking a break from work – going to the bathroom! Going to the bathroom is a totally acceptable reason for being absent from some events. You can take a work-break in the bathroom, comb your hair, retouch your make-up, and no one will question it.

An alternative solution, if the food itself really is important to you, is to allow for it in your calorie budgeting. Is this pastry more important to you than some of the food you are eating at other times of the day? Maybe you could skip breakfast to allow for it.

The third alternative is to take a low-calorie snack to work to eat at this time of temptation.

Compliments

You have been losing weight, you run into someone you haven't seen for a long time, and he or she remarks: 'Goodness – you look marvellous!'

Compliments encourage dieters but they can some-times trigger off eating temptations, too. Be aware of this! There's the temptation to decide: 'Well, if I look so good I can afford to treat myself to something extra in the way of food!'

If you are aware of this temptation you are less likely to succumb to it. But, in response to a compliment, a good motivating idea is to consider treating yourself to something that will make you look even more 'marvellous' – perhaps a new garment, hairdo or make-up experiment.

Compliments you *don't* get!

When you are doing something difficult – and shedding weight is difficult – the normal human reaction is to expect rewards for good behaviour. During a weight-loss programme, these rewards mainly come from three sources: the scales and the satisfaction of reading this tangible proof that you have lost weight; the increasing looseness of your clothes, or finding that you can fit into a smaller size; and compliments.

Compliments are very important to a slimmer.

'Goodness, you've lost weight – you *are* looking good!' We come to expect remarks like this as our weight loss starts to become obvious. What is more, we often come to depend on them. That is a little dangerous, because when we meet an old friend and *don't* get the compliment or surprised comment, it can throw us badly.

One woman recently wrote to us about a typical incident of this nature. Midway through her weight-loss campaign she was expecting an old friend to visit – a friend she hadn't seen for several months. The friend duly arrived, conversation started, but no comment was passed about the obvious weight loss.

The woman who had lost the weight had obviously been setting some store by the expected compliment; so much so that she admitted to deliberately getting up and walking across the room so that her old friend must *surely* notice!

Still no comment. . . .

Finally she was driven to ask for the compliment: 'Haven't you noticed that I've lost some weight?'

'Yes, I have,' remarked the visitor grudgingly, 'but it isn't really *you*!'

Happily, this particular incident was retrieved by a very understanding husband who quickly countered with: 'Yes, this is Margaret – it was the other, overweight person who wasn't really *her*.'

But we can't rely on someone else to make up for our disappointment. And often the disappointment at not getting a complimentary comment (let alone a sour remark!) can be strong enough to tempt us into at least a temporary dieting lapse. We haven't been rewarded for good behaviour. So we are likely to resort to bad behaviour.

There can be many reasons why we don't receive an expected compliment for our weight loss, and not all of them spring from unkind or jealous motives. Sometimes a person might have noticed that we have been in the habit of shedding a bit of weight and then regaining it. They might happen to think it more tactful not to draw attention to our efforts, lest we fail again. . . .

Sometimes even the best of our friends may overlook something about us because there is another matter on their minds. It's similar to the husband who doesn't notice his wife's new dress or hairdo, simply because his mind is preoccupied with an office problem.

Often, overweight people become so sensitive about how they look that the slightest comment or lack of comment is taken as a major assault, when it need not be.

The solution to this is constantly to look to oneself. One must learn to be able to pat oneself on the back. Counting on the people around you to provide all the rewarding feedback can be very dangerous. It's very important to be able to look in the mirror and think, 'I look better' – regardless of what anyone else seems to think.

There are times when people won't notice your appearance. Accept that fact.

There are even known instances of people having walked through New York with no clothes on – and no one having noticed *them*!

At the same time, compliments are encouraging and helpful while you are struggling to shed weight, so it isn't a bad idea to do things in order to encourage these supportive comments. Very often when slimmers have complained to us that 'no one seems to have noticed my weight loss' the reason is strikingly obvious. They are still wearing the clothes that were specially chosen to disguise their excess weight. And clothes that disguise excess weight also tend to disguise weight loss.

A pretty new blouse or a new hairdo can draw attention to appearance and attract compliments – not necessarily about your weight but about how nice you are looking. And these are pleasing and encouraging compliments too. Don't wait until you reach your target weight before starting to make the changes.

Dinner parties (your own)

Few hostesses overeat at their own dinner parties. Usually they are too busy ensuring that everyone else is well fed. Many hostesses overeat *after* their own dinner parties. To avoid the risk of having too little food for guests, it is almost inevitable that they prepare at least a little too much. And that leads to those most dangerously tempting items of food – leftovers!

If you entertain frequently, be aware that the major temptations loom when the guests have left (and swiftly turn to the sections in this book headed 'leftovers').

Eating amnesia

If you eat some little items of food when you didn't intend to eat them, you will be strongly tempted to *forget* that you ate them! This can lead to all kinds of dieting difficulties, like starting to believe that your diet plan 'doesn't work' (so what's the point in following it!) or attributing a growing weight problem to some unlikely cause like fluid and glands.

Dieticians often remark that people will never tell the truth about how much they have been eating. But our own feeling is that this is more a matter of self-induced amnesia than of 'lying'. We all have a tendency to forget things that we would rather not remember.

One dietician we know got a bit of a shock herself when she started to keep written records of everything she ate. She discovered that when she included little things like a taste of something she was cooking, or an apple, she was eating about ten times a day. She genuinely hadn't realized that she was eating so often, or eating so much! The same applies to most of us.

Keeping written records of everything you eat and the time at which you eat it is the best cure for eating amnesia. Keep a note pad handy in the kitchen, and even carry it in your handbag – because it is essential to write it down right away before amnesia has had time to set in.

People shedding weight on behavioural weight-control programmes are obliged to keep a very detailed record of everything eaten, the calorie content, and the time at which they ate it. If this sounds like too much trouble, you can at least compromise and make a brief note of what you ate and when you ate it, for example: '4 p.m. – one spoonful of the stew being cooked.'

The great advantage of the write-it-down technique, apart from curing eating amnesia, is that if you know that you are going to have to write it down you then become more tempted *not* to eat it, in order to be able to present yourself with a praiseworthy record for the day.

Eating for your feet

Very often feet tempt us to eat.

Scenario: we are having a day in town, hunting through the stores for clothes or furniture. After an hour or two our backs and feet start to ache and we want to sit down.

Have you noticed that the only seating accommodation provided in stores is in places that oblige us to buy at least a drink – and put us in close proximity to tempting food, as well? If you want to rest those feet, you've just got to head for the cafeteria or coffee shop.

You may tell yourself that you will just have a coffee. But, inevitably, the woman at the next table will be partaking of a large, cream-filled gâteau. . . . 'Oh well, perhaps just this once!'

If you have seen yourself in that situation, more than once, give some thought to your feet next time you embark on a shopping expedition or on plodding round museums with the children.

Timing the expedition to involve a natural meal-break at 'tiredness time' can help. Maybe, instead of setting off to the shops early in the morning you could start mid-morning, so that by the time you start to feel tired it's lunch time anyway, and you can carry on shopping afterwards.

If you normally eat breakfast, an alternative solution on the day of a shopping expedition would be to skip breakfast in order to allow yourself the calories for a mid-morning break wth a coffee and pastry.

It's worth noting, too, that a cocktail bar will provide less calorie-temptation than a coffee shop – as long as you sit well away from the peanuts!

Be aware that stores do not want you to sit down unless you are spending money. So they take care to ensure that you are spending money on food and drink, if not on their other merchandise. You might try getting your own back by 'testing' chairs in the furniture department!

'Eating for your feet' is a great occupational hazard for those, like nurses, who spend most of their working hours on their feet. We know of one doctor (by the name of Dr Henry Jordan, as a matter of fact) who gained twenty-five pounds in six months during his early days as a medical intern. During very long periods on his feet, calling in at the staff canteen for a meal presented the most acceptable reason for sitting down for a while, so he and his colleagues tended to take a fourth meal break during their long working day. Also, there was the temptation to help yourself to an extra course in order to prolong the rest period a little. . . .

Those whose professions involve becoming footsore and weary need to become aware that they are often eating most of the surplus calories for their feet rather than their stomach. This way they can plan how at least to limit the quantity eaten during breaks, perhaps filling up the extra gaps with extra cups of coffee.

Eating in the car

Food kept or carried in the car tempts people to eat in the car. Many of us, after loading a pile of shopping on to the front seat, have found ourselves nibbling something – particularly if it smells good – as we drive home from the shops.

Load the shopping into the back seat or boot, instead of into the front seat of the car.

Don't keep snacks in the car, because often we find ourselves sitting around in it, perhaps waiting for the children to come out of school. This puts us into a strong temptation situation – with unexpected time on our hands, and some slight feeling of boredom. It's a very good idea to keep a book or magazine in the car for moments like this.

Eating quickly

There is little doubt that if you eat your food quickly you are going to be tempted to eat more food during the course of that meal than you would if you ate slowly. What is more surprising is that you are likely to become hungry again more quickly after a rapidly eaten meal than you would if you had eaten the same quantity of food at a slower pace!

In one recent experiment people who had gobbled down a meal were actually found to produce more saliva at the sight of a snack an hour later than those who had eaten the same meal, at the same time, but more slowly.

There seems to be some definite connection between the rate of eating and the length of satisfaction, but as yet we don't fully understand the reasons.

Certainly there are many known reasons why rapid eating tempts you to overeat. Most overweight people tend to be fast eaters.

One of the more obvious reasons is that if you polish off your meal faster than do your companions at the table, you are going to be tempted to help yourself to some more food 'to keep them company'. But there are physiological reasons, too. It takes at least several minutes before the food put into the mouth has any physical effect in satisfying hunger. Fast eaters can pack down a whole load of calories in that time! It also appears to take about twenty minutes for a meal to have its maximum effect in satisfying hunger. Often people who feel just comfortable and satisfied at the end of a meal will start to feel un-comfortable and overfull about five or ten minutes later – and start to wish that they hadn't eaten so much.

Slow down. That is important advice for all weight-prone eaters. In particular, concentrate on slowing down your eating during the first five minutes of a meal because the usual pattern in meal eating is to start off at a rapid pace and then gradually eat more and more slowly as the meal progresses.

The easiest way in which to slow down is to take longer gaps between bites, ideally putting your knife and fork down between each bite. Taking smaller bites tends to be less comfortable than this procedure. People have a characteristic bite-size for different foods and the 'wrong-sized bite' feels unnatural to them.

It's a good idea to keep one eye on the slowest eater at the table and try to pace yourself to eat in time with him.

Longer and more frequent time gaps during the course of a meal also help you to eat more slowly and to eat less. If you are eating at home, serve yourself only a half portion of the dish you have cooked – then take a time gap of five to ten minutes before you go to the kitchen to help yourself to the other half. Quite often, when you start to consider it after this length of time, you will find that you no longer feel any strong *need* to finish off the dish. So you won't!

Take longer gaps between courses too. That way the next course will tend to become more resistible.

Try to make any meal last for at least twenty minutes.

This slow-down advice applies to snacks as well as meals; even to something like a bar of chocolate. The person who sits down and eats her chocolate slowly, taking gaps between bites, will gain much more eating pleasure and satisfaction out of a small quantity of chocolate and will be much less likely to binge on large quantities of chocolate.

Eating to avoid hunger

The clock tells you that it's 8 a.m. or 1 p.m. Very often, if you were really to think about it, you would realize that you weren't actually hungry. However, if you don't eat now you're sure to get the mid-morning 'sinks' or the mid-afternoon tummy rumbles . . . !

Very often we are tempted to eat not because we're hungry but in order to avoid being hungry at a later time when food might not be available.

There are some virtues in this. The snag is that we're often using up a lot of precious calories at a time when they're not really needed, and making less available for times when we're going to be yearning for them.

The best solution is a compromise. Experiment for a few days to discover how much food it really does take to satisfy your hunger for the next few hours. Often it turns out to be less than you thought. You don't have to eat a big lunch to get through to dinner without entertaining your colleagues to a tummy-rumbling symphony. You might well discover that just a little bit of food will do the trick, so this way you can save calories when it's *easy* to save them.

Eating to settle the stomach

Yuk — what's that nasty feeling going on down there? Suddenly, you become uncomfortably aware of your stomach drawing attention to itself with sharp little pains or unpleasant churning sensations. You aren't hungry, it wasn't long since your last meal, but stomach swiftly sends a message to brain: 'Eat something — then I'll feel better!'

Next time stomach strikes, *don't* eat that snack, wait a little while . . . then discover a surprising little fact. Left to its own devices your stomach can usually sort out its own problems.

It isn't just the present mild discomfort but the thought that if you don't eat to settle your stomach you will begin to feel worse that lies behind this particular temptation. In fact, nine times out of ten the discomfort doesn't get worse. Just the reverse!

The stomach is a very busy machine, constantly on the move, so it isn't surprising that at some moments it should get itself into situations which cause mild feelings of discomfort. In most cases, by carrying on moving and diluting acids, it gets itself out of those situations, unaided by an extra intake of food.

Usually, stomach discomforts are felt during unoccupied moments. Most mild sensations of pain go unnoticed when the mind is otherwise distracted. So, if you can momentarily distract your attention from your stomach, maybe by browsing through a magazine, you will often find that you forget about it, allowing it sufficient time to settle itself again.

Eating while cooking

A lot of people are tempted to eat while they cook. Not surprising, you might conclude, since the food being cooked has to be tasted! But by asking people to keep daily records of everything consumed, we have discovered that most of the food being eaten is not the food being cooked!

If the need to taste were the real problem it would be possible to follow the wine-tasters' technique of spitting it out. In fact the main problem is that most people do their food preparation prior to a meal, at a time when they are starting to feel hungry. Thus, at a vulnerable time, they place themselves in the danger area of the kitchen, close to the appetite triggers of the sight and smell of food. Not surprisingly, they are tempted to help themselves to snacks.

Decrease this temptation by preparing your next meal at the time you feel least hungry – which is after you have just eaten your last meal.

Elevators

The strongest antidote to the temptation to use the elevator, rather than walk up a few flights of stairs, is the fact that walking upstairs is one of the highest calorie-burning activities there is. It beats almost anything – except *running* upstairs!

Fat friends

Have you noticed that when *you* are trying your hardest to lose weight, your fat friends seem to be trying *their* hardest to stop you losing weight? No, you aren't imagining things. A deliberate game of sabotage is afoot. Overweight friends will often try to tempt you to break your diet with offers of food, warnings about your health – 'you're overdoing it' – reassurances that you are absolutely perfect as you are, and all the usual sabotage tactics.

You can best resist the temptations they feed into your ears (and into your mouth if they possibly can!) by understanding the true motives behind these crimes. And often the motives themselves aren't really criminal.

Overweight friends are often mainly concerned that if you change they are going to lose your friendship, and, unfortunately, that is partially true.

Overweight people sometimes stay together partly because it is comforting to be with someone else in the same situation. If your friend eats a lot, you don't feel too bad about eating a lot yourself.

As you begin to lose weight this tends to start changing the relationship considerably. Excess weight automatically places some limits on activities and interests. As you become slim you will probably become more physically active – and your overweight friend may not be able to keep up with you. If you are single you might become more interested in 'dating' activities such as going to dances and discotheques, and, again, your friend will be hesitant to share your new interests.

Your friend feels comfortable with the person with whom she has formed the friendship. It is perfectly natural for her to resist the changes that might well start turning you into a rather different person.

As you become slim you might well lose this friend and form a new circle of friendships. Don't feel frightened at this prospect, as some people do. The world doesn't end at the loss of one friend! For most people, life is a constant series of new friendships forming and old friendships dissolving. When we are single we have a certain group of friends. These tend to change when we get married, and again when we have children. Again they change if we move our home from one town to another.

Another factor that may be encouraging your friend to discourage you from losing weight is the fact that many overweight people feel some sense of guilt at not being able to reduce and control their own body weight. As you start to use self-control in eating you tend to make your overweight friend feel even more guilty. There's really nothing much you can do about that!

As you start to lose weight, expect your overweight friends to discourage you as your success starts to become apparent. Their efforts are unlikely to have any effect if you understand the motives, and are prepared for this reaction.

Fear of failure

People who are *too* fearful of failing in a slimming campaign are more likely to be tempted to give up than those who are a little less worried about it!

Psychologists have made tests to discover what degree of anxiety and concern about success is most likely to result in success. Not surprisingly, they found that those who weren't too concerned about their weight – just thought it might be a good idea to try and shed some – lacked sufficient motivation to carry on dieting during the inevitable difficult periods.

At the other extreme, those who took a fatalistic, '*this* is my last chance' attitude, and were desperately worried by the prospect of failure, were also unlikely to complete the course.

The slimmer most likely to succeed is the one who has what psychologists term 'a moderate degree of fear of failure'.

At the start of a weight-loss campaign the too-fearful person usually sheds weight very well. Her great barrier to success is the first time she breaks her diet. This often throws her into a state of panic.

Instead of deciding that she will keep on trying, she sees her first slip-up as proof of her greatest fear – she doesn't have the willpower to succeed! Often she will lapse into a guilty binge or give up dieting in despair.

To protect yourself from counterproductive, excessive fears, try to get your proportions into proportion. Your weight is important. It is not *all* important. There are other things about you that can be attractive and interesting to other people; there are things that can give you pleasure and fulfilment even if you are overweight.

And, unless your doctor happens to have given you the sternest of health warnings, there is no such thing as 'the last chance to diet'!

First courses

The first course of a three-course restaurant meal is simultaneously both the easiest and the hardest course to skip.

Were we dining alone we would usually find this the easiest course to miss, knowing that our appetites would be satisfied by the more substantial main course. Often we are not dining alone.

First courses tempt us to eat surplus calories at the start of a meal entirely because by not ordering this course we would be forced to sit and wait and watch other people eat at a time when we are feeling particularly hungry.

The tradition of eating a small savoury course before a main savoury course is, when you come to think of it, a remarkably effective temptation in causing most people to eat more food than they really want. You eat the 'extra' food because the 'extra' food comes first. Were this offered after the main course, few people would order it!

Restaurants benefit in selling more food by having a tempting array of first-course dishes on the menu.

You can turn the availability of these small courses entirely to your own advantage by following our own favourite-restaurant-food-control ploy.

Next time you are dining in a restaurant consider ordering two first courses instead of a first course and a main course. Usually you will find that you are amply satisfied by two small savoury courses. You are eating while others are eating. You don't feel deprived. And the restaurant is rendering you great assistance in portion control. At the same time you are paying less for your meal – and that's nice to know!

Far from complaining about this little eccentricity in ordering a meal, we find that dining companions, knowing that the main course usually provides more food than they need, often seize on it as an excellent idea – and follow in suit. Only the restaurant loses out. And here we are not concerned with solving their problems.

Food for thought

Recurring thoughts of food aren't just a single temptation, they are the start of almost every eating temptation. Food that comes into the mind so often ends up in the mouth.

Hundreds of little appetite triggers can start us thinking about food, particularly favourite foods that we find specially tempting. We catch a glimpse of it, somebody starts talking about it . . . suddenly that hard-to-banish recurring thought is planted firmly in the mind, and often it can intensify into a craving.

Some food thoughts are more dangerously tempting than others.

Least tempting are thoughts about food that we are going to be able to eat as part of our calorie allowance that day. The knowledge that it is only a matter of time before the desire is satisfied tends to prevent it from intensifying.

Most tempting are the thoughts of food that we aren't going to be able to eat. Those are the really dangerous thoughts that often lead to excesses.

Can you stop those thoughts? A difficult task. If there were one effective answer it would provide the overall solution to nearly all eating temptations. But psychiatrists and psychologists have been experimenting with a variety of thought-stopping techniques, which may sound a little strange, but have been found helpful for some people.

One of the simplest, recently tested with some success by psychologist Dr Edward Abramson at California State University, even involves a mild degree of torture. To 'torture yourself slim' you wear a thin rubber band around your wrist, and every time your thoughts stray to that specially tempting food you give it a sharp (Ouch!) ping.

If you still go ahead and eat the food, you punish yourself with the sting of the ping for each mouthful. Dr Abramson, using saliva-measuring tests, was actually able to measure a decreased desire to eat these tempting foods among people who put this technique to the test.

Another technique that has been tried with some degree of success is shouting 'STOP' out loud, and accompanying the shout with a vigorous physical gesture, like a clap of the hands or a thump with the fist on a table. Some people, with practice, have learned to put a stop to their own recurring food thoughts this way. Yet another technique involves imagining that you are eating those craved-for foods, but, at the same time, imagining, in somewhat vivid detail, that you are also being sick. Not one for delicate sensibilities, this!

Any of these ideas may be worth a try. A simpler method is the good old 'Don't just sit there, *do* something!' technique, because becoming mentally involved in anything else, a task or a book perhaps, can divert those dangerous thoughts. And remember, it's the thoughts of the foods you can't have which are the most dangerous. So if you can work out ways in which you can allow yourself the thought-about foods as part of your calorie allowance today, or tomorrow, you can considerably lessen this temptation.

Fragrant food shops

Self-control is best practised at the furthest distance from temptation. When you can, put physical distance between yourself and that bakery or delicatessen shop selling the foods which most tempt you – but which you aren't planning to eat as part of today's diet.

Take a detour, or cross the road. That protects you from the appetite-stimulating effect of the smell of favourite foods. If you must walk right past the shop, don't make the resolution: 'I'll just look in the window, but I won't buy.' Instead, resolve that you won't look. Aid your self-control – don't keep putting it to masochistic tests!

Goals (over-optimistic)

Most dieters show a dangerous tendency to set their weekly weight-loss goals far too high.

They do not lose as much weight as they had hoped; they are deeply disappointed. A survey on the main reasons why people break their diets put 'disappointment with weight loss' at the top of the list of temptations.

When setting up your goals it is better to put your expectations too low than too high. Choose a time period and weight-loss goal that will give you a feeling of having achieved steady progress, rather than having achieved a world speed record for weight loss! For instance, almost anyone, by plodding on with their diet, despite the occasional setback, should be able to shed two pounds in ten days. That is a comfortable and realistic kind of goal. If you reach your target you will feel pleasure. If you exceed it you will feel delighted! Both of these moods are excellent motivators for continued effort. The feeling of *not* having achieved your interim target is a very bad feeling, highly conducive to packing up your diet altogether.

Good manners (other people's)

Other people's good manners sometimes tempt you to eat more than you plan to eat by undermining the only good reason for not eating your fill.

Be aware that if you refuse food with a critical

comment about your own weight – 'No, I mustn't, I'm getting as fat as a pig!' – natural courtesy positively compels others to deny your self-criticism.

For them to say nothing indicates agreement, which would be rude. For them to agree – 'Yes, I have noticed that you have been starting to look like a pig' – would clearly be ruder.

Your well-mannered companions have no option but to protest that you aren't even the slightest bit overweight. Those with particularly good manners may even feel compelled to insist that you are verging on the underfed and emaciated. . . .

If a lot of people have been telling you that you look thin lately, it could well be because you have been telling a lot of people that you look fat.

Sometimes, because we can't form a clear picture of our own bodies (mirror image tends to get confused with 'body image' which is our often inaccurate mental picture of the way we look) we tend deliberately to criticize ourselves in order to get the reassuring feedback of denials from other people. This can temporarily lull us into a false sense of security.

Don't let your eating be influenced by other people's comments about your weight. Good manners and truth are often incompatible.

Good manners (your own)

Our own good manners sometimes tempt us to eat more than we planned, in order to avoid hurting the feelings of the person offering the food.

Most of these situations can be solved by the handy little ploy of the refusal with the built-in compliment.

A splendidly final comment to counter second-helping offers: 'That was delicious, one of the nicest meals I've had for ages – if I ate one morsel more it would spoil it!'

A tactful way to refuse unexpected offers of food: 'No, thank you, your homemade cakes are my greatest weakness – once I start I'll never be able to stop!' There are endless variations to suit all occasions.

Be more lavish with praise, and you can be less lavish in the quantity of food you accept.

Good sportsmanship

Be prepared to be a bad sport.

Once you learn to be a bad sport you will no longer feel compelled to eat the food you didn't plan to eat, and drink the alcohol you didn't plan to drink in the name of good sportsmanship.

It is patently obvious that how much food you don't eat or how much drink you don't drink cannot possibly affect the happiness of anyone else but yourself. However, people will attempt to persuade you that this is not so.

'Oh come on, don't be a spoilsport . . .' they will say, urging you to join them in a second helping of dessert.

'You're no fun,' they may complain when you say, 'No, thank you.'

It is quite amazing what many people will do in order to be considered good sports. Overweight people tend to be particularly fearful of being considered bad sports. Supersensitive about their weight, they often tend to have a low estimation of themselves and feel, incorrectly, that they have to go along with everyone else in a general attitude of 'good sportsmanship' in order to be socially acceptable.

In fact the reputation of being a good sport is a highly overrated asset.

So often it leads to the kind of attitude: 'Oh, she won't mind – she's a good sport.' Often you *do* mind the liberties perpetrated on you on this premise, but daren't say so for fear of being considered a bad sport.

Most overweight people need to learn to be more assertive, particularly in this direction.

Never eat or drink anything in order to be considered a good sport.

Don't deign to argue, protest or explain when someone is silly enough to suggest that it is unsporting to take this attitude. Fix them with an icy glare in the eyeball, and switch the conversation to something other than food.

It is unlikely that you will lose friends by showing you can't be persuaded by such silly arguments – it's much more likely that you will gain respect.

'Go on – one little piece won't hurt!'

People who tempt you with this little classic are probably right to some degree. One little piece probably wouldn't hurt in terms of excess calories. But if it's one little piece which you didn't intend to have (which is usually the case) it undermines your feelings of being in control of your food intake. That will hurt. And that's the critical issue.

This doesn't mean that you have to respond by being angry with the person who is offering the food. Sometimes they are doing it mainly out of goodness of heart. Other times there is a deliberate game of sabotage going on.

This is where you have to use some assertive behaviour, and a classic assertive technique called 'parroting' can be particularly effective. Continue to say exactly the same words over and over again: 'No, thank you, I really don't want it . . . no, thank you, I really don't want it.' Repeat for as many times as it takes. Repeating the same words several times tends to discourage the tempter more quickly than a variety of different replies and explanations.

If you give in and agree to accept the food, after refusing several times, you are setting yourself up for this same temptation to arise over and over again in the future. The food offerer will make a subconscious mental note that it takes three or perhaps four times of offering to get you to accept food. Next time you meet them in a similar situation they will automatically make the offer three or four times.

Guilt

Oddly enough, one of the strong temptations to overeat frequently arises from a resolve *not* to overeat!

Everyone overindulges in food from time to time, and for the person unconcerned about body weight this presents no real problem. Not so with the person who is determinedly trying to shed weight! Having lost control for a time, and broken a resolve, this person is often overwhelmed with a sense of guilt and self-disgust.

These feelings can be enormously strong. Patients have frequently confessed to calling themselves abusive names, dissolving into tears. . . .

Such strong regrets would, logically, put an end to further eating. In actual fact the reverse is usually the case. Any strong emotion can trigger off the desire to eat, and a strong feeling of guilt is a potent appetite trigger.

The person who feels guilty usually eats still more food to try and comfort herself, and out of a sense of failure and despair. What's the use . . . what's the point of stopping now! Weight-loss campaigns never fail because a dieter overeats at one particular meal, or on one particular day. Nearly always they come to an end because, having indulged, she feels so guilty about it that she carries on overeating.

Sometimes there is a gap between the resolve-breaking

overeating and the guilt-induced overeating which follows. The guilty person often makes an attempt to make up for her overindulgence. But usually the targets she sets for herself ('I won't eat a single thing tomorrow!') are unrealistic and unattainable, leading to an even greater sense of guilt.

To protect yourself from the counterproductive dangers of guilt, accept, right at the start of your weight-loss plan, that few people can resist every eating temptation for every hour of every day over a period of weeks or months. You are unlikely to be an exception.

In fact, if you never slipped up you would have little chance of staying slim permanently. In all learning processes, essential lessons are learned from correcting our mistakes. Regard the occasional slip-up as an integral part of learning weight control. Learn to correct it not by overcompensating but by calmly and firmly getting back into control of your eating.

Happy moods

Most people associate eating temptations with gloomy and depressed moods. In fact any kind of mood or emotion that is a little stronger than usual can trigger off a temptation to eat. This includes happy moods.

Some time ago there was a popular cigarette advertising slogan in Britain: 'Players completes the pleasure!' Smokers, on settling themselves in a hammock in the garden on a particularly sunny and happy day, are inclined to 'light up' to complete the pleasure.

In a similarly happy situation, the food-orientated person is likely to help herself to a snack to 'complete the pleasure'.

By habit we have grown to associate food with pleasure - most celebrations involve eating and drinking. One of the most important things you must learn in order to gain lasting control of your weight is that pleasure does not have to involve food and can be very complete without it. Keep reminding yourself of this, in order to resist this temptation.

Holidays

If you set off on holiday determined to ration every calorie, you are destined for a pretty miserable holiday. If you return from holiday with six or seven surplus pounds, you are destined for a pretty miserable homecoming.

Whither lies the alternative to these miseries? In compromise, we suggest. For all but the most doggedly determined, a resolve not to gain weight, or even just not to gain more than a pound or two, is more realistic than the aim of trying to shed weight amid all the obvious eating temptations of a holiday.

Two policies tend to pay off best in achieving the aim of moderation:

1. If you are staying at a hotel, book for bed-and-breakfast only, rather than paying a price to cover all your meals.

2. Make your sacrifices during the daytime hours to allow for a reasonable amount of indulgence in the evening.

Policy 1 counteracts the powerful pull of the 'I've paid for it so I *must* eat it!' temptation. Never underestimate its strength. Many of the world's greatest overeating feats have been achieved in the name of getting full value for money. We witnessed one ourselves during a Christmas hotel holiday when a fellow guest, smitten by a tropical tummy bug, was led green-faced to the table to do battle with a seven-course banquet meal. He left, eventually, greener, sicker, but triumphant! He had succeeded in consuming the banquet he had paid for as part of his Christmas holiday package deal.

An extreme case, perhaps, but most of us, however lavish with our cash and careful with our food, do feel tempted to eat the food for which we have paid. Avoid this temptation by paying for as little food as possible in advance.

Policy 2, that of saving most calories for the evening, tends to provide the best compromise between control and pleasurable indulgence. The evening meal tends to be the most important holiday meal. Dining out is often the main social activity of the evening. Often we want to sample foreign dishes and exotic foods. Concentrate on saving calories for this meal because, with this pleasure in store, you might well find it possible to skip lunch and take a swim instead, or at least to eat very little during the daytime hours.

Sometimes, if you are concerned about your weight, a moderate amount of food control on holiday actually adds to the pleasure of eating by eradicating feelings of guilt. A friend of ours experienced this during a holiday in the South of France last summer, when the pleasure of eating all that lovely French food gradually became marred by the sight of what she described as 'all those lovely little French bottoms' on the beach. Thoughts of her own somewhat more ample backview actually started to detract from her eating pleasure until she decided on a compromise policy of eating very little until the evening to 'at least stop the spread' until she could get home and diet. From then on she started to enjoy her food again.

Holidays are not only the times when we are most tempted to eat, often they are also the times when we become most aware of our figure faults. A compromise solution takes best account of both factors.

Home baking

You are alone in the kitchen. Many people are tempted to eat more when they are alone; most people are most tempted to eat when they are in the kitchen! Before you is the very tempting sight of freshly baked cakes and biscuits. Around you is the even more tempting aroma of these foods. . . .

You are now in a situation of such acute danger and temptation that you can't expect us to rescue you from it. There is, frankly, little we can do – except to urge you to bake cakes and biscuits as infrequently as possible. Bought cakes and biscuits tend to be less dangerous. If you must bake, it is better to bake large batches from time to time and store them in the freezer away from instant-nibbling temptation than to bake once or twice each week, because every time you bake you deliberately match your willpower against a quite diabolical degree of temptation.

Hostesses

On your right, your genial, generous hostess, who has gone to an enormous amount of trouble to prepare delicious food to tempt you to eat more than you intend at her dinner party this evening.

And on your left . . .?

Well, what strategies can you use to combat dishes that can hit willpower below the belt, and persuasion to second helpings that can deliver the knockout?

Generally, it isn't a good idea to try to match your willpower against the blandishments of a good hostess. So, cut down eating in advance and aim for moderation rather than deprivation if you accept an invitation.

Even then, the evening is likely to be something of a contest between you and your hostess, whose social role requires that she ensures you are amply fed. Sometimes you can disarm her in advance by a tactful warning that although you would love to accept her invitation, you won't be able to eat a large amount of food. But don't save this announcement for the dinner table. A public announcement tempts fellow guests into a bout of the entertaining sport of teasing and persuading you into breaking your diet, and only increases your number of adversaries.

In all contests, knowing your adversary helps. And often we do have a good idea of which temptations to expect from a particular hostess, because we have been entertained by her before. We might know that dinners served at this particular home are always lavish, calling for extra-strict calorie control before the feast. This may be a home where tempting hors d'oeuvres are always served at that vulnerable time before the meal, in which case, arriving a little late could helpfully cut down calories in both food and drink.

But, generally, eating and drinking slowly is your greatest safeguard against excesses. The first guests to clear their plates always receive the strongest urgings to 'have a little more'. Take care to be the last! The empty glass is a reproach to the good host or hostess. Keep yours well-filled for as long as possible by sipping slowly.

Be aware that dinner-party temptations don't always end as you wave goodnight to your hostess – particularly if you have been extra strict with yourself all evening! It is not at all uncommon, we find, for overweight people who have successfully 'struggled to resist' all evening to go home feeling so deprived that suddenly resolve cracks and they indulge in a large bout of secret eating in their own kitchens. So, remember – aim for moderation rather than deprivation on these especially tempting occasions.

Hunger

You are hungry. No one can tell you that you are not hungry because you *are*. You can actually feel it. It's not just a matter of yearning for a chocolate bar, or twitching your nose like a rabbit at the scent of those chips. You start to get that empty feeling, you start to feel uncomfortable . . . and naturally you are tempted to eat, because if you don't it's all going to get *worse*!

There's a great temptation for people to eat the moment they feel the first twinge of hunger, in order to stave off more intense feelings of hunger which will inevitably follow.

Inevitably?

Well, here's a surprising fact that our eating experiments have shown. If people delay eating for fifteen to twenty minutes after experiencing 'the first twinges', more often than not the feelings of hunger will diminish.

Hunger is a waxing and waning sensation. It does wane, though it may sometimes return again. But by experimenting with your own hunger feelings – seeing what happens when you delay eating – at least you can stop yourself being bullied by little twinges which may fade away until the next scheduled mealtime.

It's a tough fact, but in order to shed weight you may have to learn to tolerate a small degree of hunger. A nice positive thought that will help you to tolerate it is the thought of your body munching away at your own fat. Hunger is often an indication of 'negative caloric balance', which means that you are eating *you*.

Husbands (critical)

When a husband constantly nags his wife to lose weight she may diet in an attempt to please him and put an end to the criticism. This is rather a dangerous basis on which to start a weight-loss campaign. It is always a mistake to slim for someone else! If you deprive yourself for someone else you will tend to become resentful of that person – and you can never guarantee that you will achieve your goal of pleasing the other person. The temptation on achieving your object but not the expected reward is to abandon all further effort at food control.

We suspect that critical husbands are one of the main reasons why many women who have succeeded in losing weight regain it again.

There can be a variety of reasons why a husband criticizes his wife's weight. Some husbands are genuinely concerned, for the best of motives. Others may derive some comfort for their own inadequacies by constantly directing attention to what they consider to be their wives' failure.

And some husbands are just critical. A critical husband will tend to find something else to criticize once the present object of his criticism has been removed.

One patient, who had been making very good progress on her weight-loss programme, arrived at her consultation in a very angry mood: 'I've gone to all this trouble to stop him grumbling about my weight – and now the so-and-so is criticizing me for my attitude to the children,' she complained. A typical example of resentment and disappointment in this kind of situation.

Weight loss can often improve a marriage, but there is no guarantee that it will change anyone but yourself.

Don't be tempted to lose weight for someone else. The only person to lose weight for is yourself.

Husbands (helpful variety)

Quite often husbands are delighted to see that their wives are attempting to lose weight and become more attractive. Quite often they try to help. Quite often they 'help' in such a misguided way that their well-meant efforts have the opposite effect and actually tempt their wives to stop trying.

What often happens is that the supportive husband starts acting as a diet policeman and offers advice like: 'You really shouldn't have that dessert if you are trying to lose weight!' The wife interprets this as nagging and criticism, often becomes angry – may even end up eating twice as much dessert 'just to show *him*'!

The way around this problem is to choose some quiet time in the evening, maybe even after you have settled down in bed, to have a calm and non-aggressive discussion on the subject: 'Look, I know you're trying to help me and I do need your support, but some of the things that you are doing aren't helpful to me. Let me explain some of the things that would really help. . . .'

Explain that you are trying to learn to control your own eating behaviour so you don't want to be nagged because you must learn to do this yourself. Suggest some positive things your helpful husband could do which would *really* help you. Would he, for instance, mind very much if certain foods weren't kept in the house while you were dieting? Or would he mind – perhaps – if you didn't make desserts at all, because these always tempt you?

The best way to correct a well-meaning but misguided spouse is simply to discuss the question sensibly at a time when neither of you is feeling aggrieved. Don't bring it all out into the open at the moment when he has just made that infuriating suggestion, because then you will tend to sound angry and critical of his efforts.

When one partner in a marriage has a weight problem,

ıt is important for both partners to avoid direct criticism as much as possible.

Recently, at the home of some newly-married friends, we witnessed the ideal handling of a situation that could easily have led to dispute or diet breaking. The wife, who had always been overweight, had recently embarked on a dieting campaign. Among the group of friends present the suggestion suddenly came up that we should all go off to eat at an Italian restaurant. The wife, knowing that she would be tempted to break her diet if she went, but feeling tempted to go nevertheless, turned and asked her husband what he thought she should do.

His reply struck us as being the epitomy of tact: 'Well, you know that I don't mind what weight you are – but I know that it makes you unhappy when you break your diet, so maybe it's better not to go. If you don't go, I'll stay home with you, I'm not really hungry!'

Full marks for not appearing critical of his wife's weight – a very sensitive subject to her. Had he appeared to criticize it she might well have felt angry and hurt and gone out to dinner 'just to show him'! Full marks for making just a suggestion, not a decision. And full marks for giving support by offering to stay home with her.

She didn't go out to dinner!

Of course, now you have an even simpler way of dealing with that well-meaning but misguided spouse. Just leave this book open, on his bedside table, at this page!

Husbands (unhelpful)

Among the people who tempt other people to eat are husbands who insist that they prefer their wives just as they are – overweight.

It is particularly difficult to resist food if the person closest to you for most of the time is urging you not to resist it.

Sometimes a woman's own attitude is responsible. If her husband and family know that she acts as a moaning martyr when she diets, they might well shudder at the prospect, and resort to sabotage in order to restore peace and good cheer.

But some husbands have much more complex motives for resisting the weight loss of a spouse. These cases, we find, are particularly likely to occur when the wife was fat at the time of the marriage.

It is fortunate for many of us that sexual attractiveness does not necessarily conform with fashion, and a minority of men find the ample, overweight figure particularly sexually attractive. We know of some men who only ever date fat girls.

There are other men who may find excess weight emotionally attractive – seeing in the fat girl they have chosen to marry the image of someone warm, reassuring, dependable and capable.

The man who is looking for a mother replacement in choosing a wife may associate an ample figure with a maternal image. This can account for the compatibility of many married couples who seem oddly matched in a physical sense.

We can think of one married couple of our acquaintance in which this element of the relationship is strikingly obvious. He is slim and quite good looking. She is grossly overweight and looks about twice his size – and on getting to know her one finds she epitomizes the maternal figure. She is the kind of woman who always fills the house with the scents of good cooking, seems always to be surrounded by children – and sometimes scolds her husband in the same voice she uses to scold the children. He appears not to mind, and almost certainly doesn't, because on getting to know him it becomes obvious that he is the kind of man who found it easier to cope with childhood than with adult life. There is a good deal of parent-child relationship in their marriage and each satisfies the other's needs in this direction.

But another and more common reason for husbands resisting their wives' efforts to lose weight is emotional insecurity. A husband may subconsciously see the excess weight as a safety factor which will protect him from having to cope with competition, and ensure him of her continued devotion.

Many husbands feel threatened when their slimmer wives start to receive more attention from men on social occasions.

We remember one patient who received so much opposition from her husband towards her weight-loss efforts that by the time she had shed her first stone they were hardly speaking. On being persuaded to discuss the problem he eventually confessed to us that he could only think that his wife was tired of him, and wanted to make herself more attractive to other men. He even suspected that she might have found someone else already, but didn't dare ask her because he was so afraid of the answer.

There are two useful tactics for wives who face these difficult situations.

Tactic number one is to keep a low profile as a weight loser. Don't talk about it, draw as little attention as possible to your dieting efforts. Fortunately, weight loss is a gradual process giving those around us time to adjust their attitudes gradually. And people tend not to notice gradual changes unless their attention is drawn to them. It is always the acquaintance you haven't seen for a long time who will remark: 'My goodness – haven't you changed, haven't you lost weight!' The people who see you every day are much less aware of the change.

Tactic two is obviously to reassure the insecure husband

with attention and affection. This gradually helped to solve the problems of the patient we mentioned.

Resistance to the weight loss of a spouse is often based more on 'what might happen' than on what actually happens. Often we find that a husband who tries to discourage his wife from dieting changes his attitude completely when he finds himself with a slim wife who does *not* rush off and leave him as he had feared! Husbands like this are often delighted with the result of the weight-loss campaign.

It is unwise to let a marriage partner discourage you from dieting because you never can tell how that attitude might change. The only way to find out is to go ahead (unobtrusively) and work at getting slim.

Ice-cream

Ice-cream is one of the most ever-present foods of this age. It's in many people's homes, on all restaurant menus – one of the few foods that can actually approach you on the tray of a cinema usherette or the mobile kiosk of a street vendor.

Why did you eat that ice-cream?

To this question the repentant ice-cream eater could often, with honesty, give the same reply as the man who was asked why he climbed Everest: 'Because it's there.'

Ice-cream really isn't such a bad thing in terms of calories. Because it is a light, frozen foam, a moderate portion tends to provide less calories than most other desserts. The thing to guard against is a lot of ice-cream. Because of its easy availability, between meals as well as at meals, many people are tempted to eat large or frequent servings.

Large family packs kept in the home provide the strongest temptation – here many dieters have developed a cunning little tactic in order to fool themselves. Not wanting to succumb to a portion of ice-cream they decide on 'just a spoonful', and dip a spoon straight into the large container. Frequent and usually fast-forgotten dips like this can add up to a large number of ice-cream calories in the course of a day.

If you are strongly tempted by ice-cream it is best to avoid keeping a large family pack in the home. Individual-portion packs demand a more definite decision before they are opened – and are less likely to be the cause of mindless nibbling.

One of the main dangers of ice-cream is that it is a food that can be demolished very rapidly – and fast eating always tends to lead to large quantities. To correct this problem we particularly commend the virtues of the ice-cream cone. By consuming your ice-cream lick by lick you will take considerably longer to finish it than you would if you ate it from a spoon. A small portion licked from a cone provides a lengthy period of eating satisfaction which helps to negate the desire for more – and the danger of eating too much ice-cream.

'If I eat a bit I'll eat a lot'

Some dieters take this attitude to their most irresistible foods. They decide that they won't even have a taste of the stuff, for fear that it will trigger off a binge.

That's fine – if it works! We do recall one patient who resolved never to eat his own personal 'food Salome' again – ice-cream – *and* he didn't. But he is warmly remembered for being something of an exception to the general rule.

Usually, sooner or later, you are going to come up against your own least resistible food at a moment when your resistance is at its lowest ebb. Someone is going to offer you cheesecake or chocolate or chips when you are feeling hungry, fed-up or generally disillusioned with your own diet campaign.

There are such things as self-fulfilling prophecies and the attitude, 'If I eat a bit I'll eat a lot' is usually a self-fulfilling prophecy which tempts people into eventually binging on their favourite foods. If you strongly believe that you will lose all food control once you start eating this food then it's ten to one that you *will*!

For this reason it is much better to take the attitude that you will avoid your favourite food as much as possible than to tempt yourself into a future binge with that somewhat unrealistic resolve: '*I shall never eat this again!*'

If you are particularly worried about your ability to stop once you have started eating certain foods, you should deliberately practise eating small quantities of those foods at times when your appetite is well under control, in order to banish self-fulfilling 'fears of the inevitable'.

'I'm buying this for *them*'

By far the most common reason for those foods which you are trying to avoid as much as possible finding their way into your house to tempt you is: 'I'm buying these for the family.'

Without wishing to be in any way bossy or critical, we would like to persuade you to discover how much of this food – biscuits, perhaps – is being eaten by you and how much is being eaten by *them*. Ideally, keep a written record of how many of those biscuits were consumed by you.

Some of our patients who've tried this have got a bit of a shock! Quite often they have discovered that the score worked out something like two-thirds to me, one-third to them.

Sometimes, overweight people will find that their families aren't really too bothered when they cease buying certain tempting foods. They will discover that they were actually buying these foods mainly for themselves. Another point to consider is whether you are really doing your children a favour by regularly supplying them with tooth-rotting foods, rather than buying them only as an occasional treat.

Honesty is good for the figure.

Impulse food-buying

To protect yourself against impulse food-buying, which tempts you into impulse eating, never go shopping without a shopping list. Prepare your shopping list when you are not feeling hungry. Resolve, firmly, that you will buy *only* the foods on the list, nothing more. This is your greatest safeguard against the lure of those luscious food displays which are specially designed to tempt you into impulse buying.

Insults

No one actually enjoys being insulted, but there is little doubt that most overweight people have an even greater sensitivity to insults than others – particularly insults directed in any way at that greatest area of sensitivity, their weight. Even remarks which weren't intended to be insulting are construed as such, and cause deep pain.

Sometimes, insulting remarks can motivate a weight-loss campaign: many people can cite a certain comment which acted as 'the last straw' and led to positive action. But, just as often, a hurtful remark can lead to a feeling of hopelessness and the temptation to turn despairingly to food for comfort. There can even be a degree of subconscious self-punishment in this form of eating.

'So I went home and cried and cried and then I just ate and ate . . .' is a remark we have often heard from people who have suffered from these situations.

One woman who experienced this reaction was a heavily overweight thirty-year-old who came for help after responding to an insult in a way which considerably shocked her – and more than startled the people around her!

Like most heavily overweight people, she had been silently suffering personal comments about her weight for years, until, walking along a busy shopping street one day, she overheard a passer-by commenting to a friend: 'Just look at that great fat woman!'

Suddenly, in response to this 'last straw' insult, our heroine reached breaking point and put her full weight into action. Swinging back her handbag, she brought it full-force around the head of the passing commentator.

Then she ran home, as fast as her weight would allow, where she cried and cried and then ate and ate . . .

Dwelt on over the next few days this personal crisis eventually brought her to the decision that no amount of food was worth that amount of misery, and that was when she resolved to tackle her surplus weight.

But the unusual aspect of this story is that, in response to an insult, this woman did something. Most overweight people do nothing.

One of the reasons why people make 'jokes' or insensitive comments about other people's weight is that overweight people will usually go to enormous efforts to hide the fact that they do find these comments insulting. The sudden violence of the handbag attack resulted from the build-up of years of suppressed emotions.

If you deal with an insult at the time, you will be less likely to try to deal with it afterwards, by eating. But you must use the right method of dealing with it – the method which switches the embarrassment away from yourself and back to the person who made the insensitive remark. This involves assertive rather than aggressive behaviour.

Most insults centred on weight result from a lack of sensitivity rather than a deliberate wish to hurt. They are best dealt with by a simple statement of your true feelings.

Next time someone comments on your weight, discover the simple effectiveness of telling the truth by responding: 'I find that remark very hurtful.' Then the perpetrator will squirm, apologize and look for a hole in which to sink. No one likes to be made to realize that they have been insensitive, tactless or cruel.

Avoid silent suffering, and avoid the opposite extreme of trading insult for insult, which inevitably leaves two people feeling upset and undignified. The warm satisfaction of having dealt with an insult with dignity can do more than anything else to rob it of its sting!

'I thought *you* were supposed to be dieting!'

When one of your near ones, dear ones, or friendly ones has the nerve (and they're almost sure to!) to make this remark as you deliberately help yourself to the carefully planned and controlled portion of cake that you have budgeted for as part of your calorie allowances, you are going to face another unexpected temptation: the temptation to eat the whole damned cake – just to show 'em! – the temptation to feel so infuriated that you lose all eating control.

The problem arises partly because of a tendency common in overweight people to eat certain foods – the foods that have been widely identified (often incorrectly) as being particularly fattening – only in private. Many overweight people feel self-conscious about eating sugary or starchy foods when others are watching.

We recall one woman confessing that in her overweight days she used to eat biscuits in large quantities, but could never bring herself to let her husband or her children see her eating them. She would sneak down into the kitchen in the night, and sit eating biscuits in the dark rather than risk being found out. Behaviour like this is common among people who are sensitive about their weight.

In modern dieting the emphasis has moved away from banning certain foods. The emphasis is moving towards stricter fat control, and more freedom with carbohydrate foods – which, in some instances, do not deserve their fattening reputation.

To protect herself from being infuriated out of eating control by other people's old-hat ideas of what she should and shouldn't be eating, the person who is working at shedding weight needs to come out into the open. Use some assertive behaviour to shed shyness about eating *any* foods in public, and explain clearly to those around you what foods you will be eating during your weight-loss programme.

Explain to your family at the start of your slimming campaign that your calorie allowance does permit you to eat a certain amount of certain foods that they might consider to be 'indulgent' – and that henceforth they will be seeing you eating these foods as part of your weight-loss plan. At the same time it might be wise to explain, with tact, that it will be none of their business whether you are eating these foods as part of your diet or in the form of an occasional lapse. Generally, home-based 'calorie police-men' are more likely to infuriate you into eating more, rather than restrain you into eating less!

When the 'I thought *you* were supposed to be dieting' comment crops up in a restaurant, the best response is: 'It's OK, I've allowed for this as part of my calorie allowance for the week.' Just a simple statement. No need to be over-aggressive or over-defensive.

Kitchens

Your kitchen is the prime danger zone, presenting you with more eating temptations than almost any other place in the world.

For this reason we are very anxious to keep you out of your kitchen!

This isn't always easy, because in many homes the kitchen is a social centre, a cosy conversation centre, a hobby centre, a relaxation centre . . . Literally hours of the day are spent within hands' reach of food, and often amid the appetite-tempting aroma of food being cooked.

We once had a patient whose food records showed an unusually high frequency of eating – she was snacking, we discovered, as frequently as every thirty minutes throughout the day and evening. Although some overweight people will say that they are 'eating all the time', most, we find, experience some lengthy periods relatively free from food temptation during the average day. Not so in the case of this girl!

Eventually we began to locate the cause of this non-typical behaviour. This patient, we discovered, virtually lived in her kitchen. Her desk, her favourite rocking-chair and her hi-fi set were in the kitchen. Whatever she was doing, whether studying (she was a student) or relaxing, she was in close proximity to food.

The only solution was to get her out of that kitchen, and at first she proved somewhat resistant to the move. But gradually we persuaded her to ease her way out, first by moving her rocking-chair and hi-fi to another room, then her desk, followed by the telephone (also in the kitchen, we discovered!). She had to convince herself, step by step, of the benefits achieved in eating control, before reluctantly vacating her favourite den.

As a result of this experience, all patients are now asked

to make a detailed list of everything not related to food preparation which they keep in the kitchen – and all the reasons which take them in and out of the kitchen during the course of a normal day.

In many homes people go in and out of the house through the kitchen door, or let pets in and out through the kitchen door, keep telephones and even television sets in the kitchen, use that handy kitchen table for paying bills, writing letters and shopping lists . . .

Write out your own list. Then work at eliminations. Every time you go into your kitchen you are putting yourself in close proximity with food – and temptation.

Kitchen counters

Many people leave temptation lying around on the kitchen counter in the form of transparent jars, through which foods like biscuits and dried fruit can shout: 'Eat me!'

Almost as bad are tempting foods kept in non-transparent containers on the kitchen counter. These flash messages like: 'I am a cake tin, inside are cakes, eat one!'

No harm in keeping non-snackable foods, like flour, on open display. But put a cupboard door between you and snack foods to decrease kitchen eating urges.

Leftovers after visitors

While we are struggling to shed weight, visitors coming to our home often provide us with an excellent excuse to cook the foods we are tending to avoid because we find them so tempting. Here's an excellent, personally acceptable reason to bake that cake or make those biscuits! Here's a great temptation to eat much more of them than we ever estimated.

The common tendency in catering for visitors is to overestimate rather than underestimate the quantity of food that will be required. No one wants to risk not having sufficient food to offer.

What this usually leaves us with after the visit is leftovers of a particularly tempting nature. What we usually do is consume them ourselves – eating much more surplus food after the visitors have left than while we were eating with them.

One excellent solution to this problem, which will test your willpower but enhance your reputation as a generous hostess, is to offer the leftover food to the visitors to take away: 'We'll never eat all this – won't you take some home for your family?' Or with understanding friends you might be perfectly honest and say: 'If this cake is left in the kitchen I'll be tempted to eat it – and I'm trying to lose weight. Would you like to have it?'

An alternative solution for those with home freezers would be to freeze the food so that at least it is safe from instant-nibbling urges.

Leftovers (large)

When a reasonably large quantity of food is left over after a meal, it can tempt you to keep helping yourself to a little bit more and a little bit more for the next few hours – even the next couple of days – *unless* you make an immediate aftermeal decision on what you are going to do with it.

There are a variety of things you can decide to do with leftover food when there is sufficient quantity to provide another meal for one person or for the whole family. If you own a freezer, you can decide to freeze it so that it is unavailable for instant-nibbling, but can be used for a meal in the future. If you plan simply to put it in the refrigerator, decide how and when you are going to use it up. Will you serve it as part of the family supper tomorrow, or eat it for your own lunch, or what?

The thing *not* to do is to put it in the refrigerator with no firm notion of how and when you are going to use it up. That way you usually end up eating it yourself in the form of surplus between-meal snacks.

Leftovers (little)

Little portions of leftover food often provide an even greater temptation to snack than large quantities of leftover food. People have a habit of putting little pieces of pie or other small quantities of leftover food into dishes and popping them into the refrigerator.

What are you going to do with that little bit of leftover food?

It isn't large enough to provide another meal, or even another dessert. It's going to lie around in the refrigerator for a while, and sooner or later – almost certainly – as you keep noticing it, you are going to end up eating it as an extra snack, in an impulsive moment, and not as part of your overall eating plan. Little bits of leftover food lying around in the refrigerator simply call out to be eaten.

The only sensible thing to do with little bits of food left over after a meal is to throw them away. And throw them away *immediately* after a meal.

Better still, get someone else to throw them away. In any family with children aged seven or over it would be very reasonable to allocate to them the task of clearing the table and scraping the plates. It isn't at all a bad idea to explain to the children that by doing this for you they will be helping you in your slimming efforts. It is in areas like this that members of the family can give real support to a person trying to lose weight.

Many people find it very difficult to throw food away. They have to overcome a real psychological barrier in forcing themselves to recognize that there are occasions when the most sensible thing to do with food is to throw it away. Thoughts of 'wicked waste' and 'the starving in India' overwhelm their logical reasoning.

Logical reasoning will clearly indicate that a little portion of leftover pie cannot be parcelled up and posted off to India. Neither will the fact that that portion of pie is in your stomach, rather than in the garbage bin, help anyone in India. Neither will it help you – just the opposite. If you are rightly concerned about the under-nourished of the world, there are constructive ways of helping them. Eating up all those little leftovers is not one of those constructive ways. So, if no one else wants it, and it isn't big enough to provide another meal, throw it away.

Mindless eating

'Mindless' eating almost inevitably leads to *more* eating. An odd fact, indeed, but then eating behaviour is an odd and complex subject.

Our research reveals that most people feel the urge to fill two food quotas during the course of an average day. There's a physical quota, requiring sufficient food to satisfy the stomach. There's a psychological quota, too, requiring sufficient food to provide pleasure and relaxation.

When food is eaten while the mind is distracted it fails to contribute towards the second quota. Hence the temptation to eat more food!

Typical situation: a young mother is eating her own lunch while spooning food into the mouth of her baby. Distracted by the baby, she gives little thought to her own eating until the baby is fed and settled down. *Then*, so often, she sits down and helps herself to another snack to provide the pleasure and relaxation that was missing from the meal.

Food eaten while the mind is absorbed by a television programme, a film, a newspaper, a task, means mindless eating. And each mindless morsel is usually matched by an extra morsel, maybe hours later, consumed to fill that daily satisfaction quota. When you eat without thinking about what you are eating, it is almost as if you just haven't eaten at all!

Our research shows that mindless eating often accounts for almost half the calories that many people consume in a day. What a shocking waste of food! What a wasteful way to pile up extra calories!

Switch off the television, put down that newspaper; and when you eat, give full pleasurable attention to that food. This needn't mean supping in solitary silence. For most people, a background of music or radio or family conversation (as opposed to earnest business conversation) provides just sufficient diversion to encourage leisurely eating without distracting the mind from the pleasure of the food.

Mother

When she sees you undereating – even though you are doing this deliberately for your own good – your mother will usually try to tempt you to eat.

Yes, you've probably noticed! Those gifts of food. That favourite cake specially baked for your visit. Those 'don't you think you're overdoing it' remarks.

The urge to feed offspring is a strong part of the maternal instinct. And once a mother, always a mother. Even though you are an adult, your mother will still respond to you as a mother, and to some degree you will still tend to respond as if you were a child. Often, a sixty-year-old woman will still respond in a child-like way to her eighty-year-old mother.

It is very difficult for a mother to give up her mothering role as she gets older. She still needs to be a mother – and often she will seek to fulfil this need by continuing to act as a food provider, playing what part she can in ensuring that you are 'properly fed', just as she did when you were a little child.

This won't apply only to you. She will tend to react to your children in the same way, and want to feed them too.

We recall one typical problem experienced by an overweight patient with children of her own, whose own mother lived with her. The grandmother had a terrific need to buy, and bring into the home, food for her grandchildren. Unfortunately, a large part of the food being brought to the grandchildren was being consumed by their mother.

Our patient didn't feel she could ask her mother to break this habit without hurting her feelings. Finally, an alternative solution was worked out, which would take into account the needs of the grandmother as well. It was suggested to the grandmother that she take the children out for an ice-cream once or twice a week as a special treat, rather than buying them other food treats. This resolved the problem happily.

Sometimes, perhaps by making calorie savings in advance of a visit to your mother's home, it is possible to make a compromise between her needs and your own.

Often, however, we have to encourage overweight people to be somewhat assertive in requesting their mothers not to bring food or provide food during visits.

A full explanation to your mother of how she can help you to solve your weight problem by not bringing you or serving you with tempting food is best made *not* when she has just put an array of food before you. That is the time when the food being offered is most likely to become an issue and lead to hurt feelings. Much better to give your explanation in advance of this kind of situation arising.

'My doctor has told me to lose weight' can be an effective comment which most mothers will find difficult to ignore.

Office celebrations

Someone is leaving, someone is getting married, someone is having a birthday . . . ! In most offices those celebration cakes are offered around frequently – not just occasionally.

These are not rare and unique happenings. They are a regular part of office life, and can crop up as often as once a week or once a fortnight in large offices. Recognizing this puts you on the right path to coping with this temptation. It cancels out that common diet get-out clause: 'Ah, but this is a unique occasion when my normal rules needn't apply.' It gives you an opportunity to plan in advance. What are you going to do when the cake is offered around? It will be!

There are many different ways of handling this situation. Probably the worst way is to opt out of the celebration completely, because office life involves friendships and socializing and you don't need to miss out on these pleasures. In fact, few people will take offence if you decline the food and simply congratulate them warmly on their engagement or whatever the cause of celebration – maybe raise a glass of low-calorie cola in their honour!

Overweight people have a tendency to avoid drawing attention to themselves. They don't wish to make an issue of the fact that they are overweight and can't eat everything freely. They tend also to have a greater than average fear of giving offence. When they learn to say, 'No, thank you' (not only to food, but in other areas of life), they are often pleasantly surprised to discover that many people don't take issue.

Sometimes, of course, the food offerer will go into the 'Go on, just this once won't hurt' routine. If you have decided to say, 'No, thank you' on these occasions, you may have to say it several times on the first occasion. But the persuasion will decrease on subsequent occasions as people begin to realize that you really mean it.

A useful lie: 'I'd really love to – but my doctor has told me I mustn't.' Few people will feel comfortable in persuading you to go against doctors' orders.

An alternative way of dealing with this temptation is to accept the food, but only a small portion. A token morsel. If a whole large cake is being offered around, you can ask to cut your own slice. In the case of individual cakes maybe you can choose a small one or suggest sharing it with another dieter in the office.

The third alternative would be to assess, from past experience, how often these occasions tend to happen in your particular workplace. Then allow for eating this once-a-week or once-a-month cake as part of your overall calorie plan.

Maybe you can think out other ways of coping with this office temptation. The important thing is to think about it, recognize that it *will* happen, and plan in advance.

Office snack bars

In many offices and workplaces this is where you and your friends go every day for an inexpensive and convenient lunch. Usually the choice of meals is limited, and often there aren't many or even any choices that are low in calories.

There are a number of alternative ways of handling this temptation.

You could decide not to go to the cafeteria at all – and, instead, take a packed lunch and sit behind your desk to eat it. That is a slightly drastic solution because it removes many of the advantages of taking a lunch break – you miss talking to your friends, and moving away from the work environment into a more relaxed pleasurable environment.

The second alternative is to take your own packed lunch, and eat it in the cafeteria – most cafeterias will allow this – in the company of your friends, just ordering a beverage. This way you can control your food without losing your company.

A happy compromise is sometimes to take your own lunch, but at other times to order meals from the cafeteria when low-calorie meals are available. Most cafeteria menus are planned well in advance. Often it is easy enough to ask and find out what will be on the menu for the remainder of the week.

An excellent idea in a big office and if you can get enough weight-conscious friends together is to go to the cafeteria manager and say: 'Look, there are thirty of us here who are concerned about our weight – would it be possible to put something on the menu each day for us?'

In some offices, lunches are provided free of charge. We have actually had occasional letters from overweight people pointing out that they *have* to eat a cafeteria lunch 'because it is free'. Any reasonable person will clearly see that to eat surplus calories which will make you fat and miserable, simply 'because they are free', verges on insanity.

Open buffets

Why is it that by the time we reach the end of the buffet

table we so often find our plate piled up with much more food than we intended to get? In consequence we eat so much more than we intended. (No one wants to appear 'greedy' by helping themselves to more food than they can consume!)

Well, there's an immediate temptation, as we start at one end of the table, to help ourselves to the first foods that meet our eyes. Who knows what's going to be at the other end of the table – it may not be so good!

As we proceed along the table we see even more tempting foods. So we keep adding those to the plate. By the time the end of the table is reached that plate is piled very high.

To avoid this situation the best ploy is to go up to the open buffet and deliberately walk from one end of the table to the other before picking up a plate. See what's there and make some decision about which foods you really most want to eat. Then pick up a plate and select only those choice items of food.

You are now going away from the table with less food but with the option to go back for more if you wish. That provides a second decision point – whether to go back for second helpings. Often you will decide that you have really had enough. The buffet will no longer seem quite so tempting now that you are no longer so hungry.

If the table array includes some foods which look intriguing – but you're not sure whether you'll like them or not – serve yourself only very small portions of these foods so that you can try the taste and decide whether to have more.

Parking

Car parks are too close to most of the places we visit. They tempt us *not* to burn calories in the form of activity. And weight control depends on calorie expenditure as well as on calorie intake.

What is more, most of us will go to considerable trouble to locate the 'closest' place in the too-close car park. Sometimes we will drive round for several minutes, or wait for other cars to move, in order to park at the place nearest to the store entrance. Generally, much more time is spent in looking for the nearest-to-the-door spot than would be spent in walking from a more distant place in the car park to the store.

We must admit to having indulged in this illogical activity ourselves in the past. We are now reformed – and hope that you will reform too!

That short walk might seem irrelevant in terms of calorie expenditure. But most people can significantly increase their overall calorie expenditure by being more active in lots of little ways as part of their everyday activities.

Overweight women tend to be very resistant to the idea of what they consider to be 'exercise'. They often feel embarrassed at the thought of being seen rushing around a tennis court. But just walking is an excellent calorie-burning exercise. If you are overweight you gain the advantage of burning more calories than the slim person in moving your body from place to place.

For most overweight people, increased activity is best approached on a literally step-by-step basis. Start by parking your car at the most distant spot in the car park. Then progress to parking at a more distant car park, so that you are walking at least part of the way. Buy a shopping basket on wheels so that when shopping you don't have to park near the shops due to the prospect of staggering back with a difficult load. Eventually you may reach the stage when you walk all the way to the shops and don't take the car out at all. Such changes in habit *will* have a lasting and significant effect in helping you to control your weight.

Work at resisting all those modern-day temptations not to walk.

Partners in dieting

Enthused with the idea of starting a slimming campaign, many people have a tendency to encourage a friend or relative to join them: 'Let's do it together!' There are hidden dangers in this situation. Unexpected temptations can arise.

Usually, at the outset when the enthusiasm is very high, this is a very motivating kind of alliance to have. But almost universally, in a weight-loss programme people progress at different rates, or people run into different situations which throw them off for a while.

Often, the person doing least well will begin to feel somewhat frustrated and envious, and, more surprisingly, we find that the person doing well often starts to feel a little guilty.

There is a strong likelihood that the person doing least well will at some stage drop out. Then, if the other partner has placed importance on the 'joint alliance', she is going to be strongly tempted to drop out too.

Right at the outset of a joint slimming campaign it is important to realize that if you are the person who has suggested slimming, you are likely to be the person with the strongest motivation. The decision to lose weight has to be a very deliberate decision, and a very individual decision. You can't completely persuade anyone else to make that decision – although they may seem to agree with it in the first flush of enthusiasm. For this reason, if you suggest a joint slimming campaign to a friend or relative, it's an excellent idea to ask them to think about it for twenty-four hours before making a decision.

Even then, it is very important to accept, right at the

start, that your progress and success must not become dependent on the other person's progress and success. Don't attach your success in weight loss to whether or not somebody else is doing well. You have made a personal decision to shed weight. If somebody else shares the trials and triumphs with you, that will be great – and helpful. But if they fail, this must not be allowed to provide an excuse for you to fail as well.

Another hidden danger of a slimming-together campaign: we have known instances of friendships breaking up when one person succeeds and the other fails. Here one has to make a personal decision – is my weight loss, and the advantages that weight loss will give me, more important to me than the loss of this particular friendship? Or perhaps just the temporary break-up of this particular friendship?

Generally, in seeking support in your slimming, it is safer to team up with a group rather than one individual. In a group you will always find some members whose attitudes will continue to support your own motivation. With an individual it is much more risky.

Resist the temptation of taking a 'we sink or swim together' attitude if you are slimming with a friend. Rather, take the attitude – even if she sinks, I'll continue to swim. And slim!

Peanuts

The big problem for peanut addicts is not that one peanut inevitably leads to another peanut; it is that one *handful* of peanuts inevitably leads to another handful of peanuts. And another.

If peanuts are your temptation, never eat them out of the bag or can in which you buy them. We all have a tendency to finish up a whole unit of food. If you start eating from the bag, it's ten to one that you won't finish until the bag is empty.

If you *do* buy peanuts (after seriously considering the alternative of not buying them at all!), pour a small quantity out of the bag into a small dish. Take the small dish, not the bag, to your designated eating place.

If you *do* buy peanuts, it is far, far better to buy them in their shells than shelled. This way you will probably buy less, you won't be able to eat them by the handful, you will be forced to eat them much more slowly, and will inevitably end up eating less peanuts.

If you *don't* buy peanuts but find bowls of them thrust before your eyes at parties, the sensible thing is to station yourself well away from the peanuts. If you have to make a small journey in order to obtain another handful, your natural sense of decorum (and wish not to appear greedy) will automatically ration your intake.

Persistent cravings

You have to learn to say 'No' to yourself when you are trying to shed weight. If you continue to give in to every little impulse to eat everything you fancy, your shadow is likely to increase rather than lessen.

But with cravings for specific foods, fighting for *too* long a period can be dangerous. It can result in the knock-out of a binge rather than in just losing points by overeating a little.

Many cravings will disappear with a little firm handling, especially if you distract your mind with some activity rather than just sitting there thinking about that particular food.

But other cravings can be nasty, persistent things. If you fight a craving all day then wake up next morning *still* craving for that particular food, it is usually better to satisfy that craving with a small quantity than to let the craving intensify to the stage where you lose all control and dive into a large quantity.

We recall one young woman telling us about a particularly lengthy contest she held with a chocolate éclair. One morning, driving home after delivering her children at school, she just happened to notice an especially delicious-looking éclair in a bakery window. She thought about that éclair on and off for the rest of the day. The next day she passed the shop again and her cravings for the éclair became even more intense throughout that day. On the third morning, still thinking of the éclair, she stopped her car at the shop, bought an éclair – just one, not half a dozen – took it home and ate it in a slow and controlled way as part of her lunch. The moment she had had the éclair the craving disappeared.

They usually do if they are satisfied in this deliberate and well-controlled way without feelings of guilt.

If this young woman had persisted in her determination not to eat the éclair, then felt furious with herself when she finally succumbed and went into the shop, the chances are that she would have bought half a dozen éclairs (telling herself that most of them were for the family) and then gone home and gobbled the lot.

Potato chips

Not only opportunities are golden. Some temptations are golden too!

Potato chips. When did you last leave a single chip on a plate? Don't feel badly if you can't remember, because we can't remember either. There's something specially tempting about potato chips, there's something even more tempting about that last one. It may not be the last chip in the world but there's something singularly precious about it.

So, while part of learning wise eating behaviour lies in learning to leave a little, you might find this task too difficult when it comes to chips.

The best time to control your temptation to eat too many chips is before they actually get on to your plate.

There is nothing even the slightest bit tempting about a cold little finger of raw potato. A golden succulent-smelling chip is highly tempting. When you are cooking chips for the family, give careful thought to the quantity you prepare before they are detonated into danger items by that hot fat.

If you cook just enough to provide an adequate portion for everyone else and a small portion for you, it's going to be pretty difficult for you to indulge in a large portion. That could lead to a family riot!

Certainly, after eating your modest portion of chips you have the option of going back to the kitchen and cooking some more if you are still tempted to eat more. But this involves a definite decision and quite a lot of time and trouble. It is unlikely that you are going to take up that option.

Potato-chip-eating temptations don't only arise in the home. They lurk in every fast-food restaurant. You have several options in coping with the ready-made chip. You could decide to skip these places altogether. If you step inside in company with other eaters, you may decide not to order chips for yourself – but to pinch a few from someone else's plate. For some people, 'just a few' will largely satisfy the taste and desire. Another option, if you are with another weight-prone person, is to order one portion between two people so that you satisfy the desire while limiting the quantity.

Pouring your own

'But I only had *one* . . .!'

When you only have one whisky, gin or other alcoholic drink in the bar, the barman can be counted on to control the quantity for you. When you pour your own at home, here's a splendid opportunity (and temptation!) to bask in the virtue of having 'only one or two' drinks — blissfully unaware that you may have poured down two or three hundred calories in the process.

The size of your glasses can help to control this temptation. A large glass encourages us to pour more, whether it is alcohol or other calorie-supplying drinks. A *wide* glass makes more look less! A small narrow glass provides the greatest restraint to your personal generosity.

Quite possibly you would find the idea of carefully measuring every drink you pour a bit of a bore. If so, at least do an initial test to get your eye in on estimating how many calories you are pouring. Using the glasses you will normally use at home, measure out one fluid ounce, two fluid ounces etc. of your favourite alcoholic drinks (noting the calories per ounce) and take a close look at how far those quantities measure up in your own glasses.

Premenstrual food cravings (Big T!)

For many women this is Big T: the major temptation which causes them to binge, break their diets and go somewhat berserk in eating. We estimate that at least one out of every three women experiences very strong food cravings for a period of three or four days prior to the start of the monthly menstrual period.

This very potent biological force is no respecter of persons nor even of well-established 'good eating habits'.

Often, when we lecture to dieticians or other experts involved in giving diet advice, there will be a great sign of personal identification when this problem is raised.

Premenstrual food cravings probably largely account for the fact that, for women, the time at which that very determined dieting campaign is most likely to fall apart is after about three weeks.

We don't fully understand the reason why these biological and psychological eating urges come into effect at this time of the month. Certainly there is no known medicinal cure. Diuretics don't help – because it is more likely that the biological factors are linked to insulin levels than to fluid levels in the body.

The nature of these food cravings varies between different individuals. Some women get them like clock-work, at the same time of the month, every month; others find that sometimes they happen and sometimes they don't. For many women the problem will centre around intense cravings for some specific foods – it can be anything under the sun. Others will experience the urge to eat anything and everything on a very continual basis during this time.

We don't have one pat solution to Big T. But if you suffer from this problem, there are ways in which you can certainly prevent it from being a major cause of weight gain, or cause of death to your latest dieting attempt!

The most important thing is to *recognize* this problem, and to be aware of when it is likely to occur. If you are the kind of woman who forgets when she had her last period and when the next one is due, start keeping a note of it in your diary. And make a note, too, of the days on which you experienced your strong premenstrual eating urges – then you will know when they are next likely to occur.

This problem is, in fact, extremely time-limited. It helps a lot just to recognize that fact. You are unlikely to become overweight simply from overeating for three or four days every month. And, when you come to think about it, there is no reason to decide that you can't diet successfully just because you may be unable to diet during just three or four days out of every month.

It's really the after-effects of this problem that are the main cause of weight gain or diet demise. You tend to feel so shattered that you have eaten so much for the past three or four days that you carry on overeating to comfort yourself. Or you decide that you are a hopeless dieting flop and that there is no point in making any attempt to carry on dieting. You have made such a thorough job over the past days of breaking every dieting rule that you obviously lack any willpower at all!

So calm down – and get this problem in its correct time-limited perspective!

There are various ways in which you can attempt to limit the number of calories consumed at Big T time. There is a particularly good one if you are one of the many women who experience cravings for specific foods.

We had one patient whose premenstrual cravings centred around biscuits. In no way could she curb the urge to eat them. The advice given to her: then try eating biscuits *instead* of some of your meals!

She tried this – and succeeded in demolishing twelve biscuits for lunch one day. However, normally she would have had lunch and then demolished about twelve biscuits during the course of the afternoon, so at least she had saved the calories which she would usually have eaten in the form of a lunch which she didn't particularly crave. She found that by substituting craved foods for meals she had less calories than she would normally have eaten during these difficult days, and although she didn't lose weight, she didn't gain any.

The thought of eating biscuits or chocolate instead of those nutritious mealtime foods might strike you as being very sinful. However, you won't become malnourished or experience an outbreak of scurvy from eating in this way for just three or four days every month! No nutrients are required on a daily basis, and if you get the right average quantity of vitamins, minerals and protein over a period of weeks, you won't come to any harm.

If you are following a diet and badly want to avoid 'losing ground' for any reason at all, you might try banking extra calories for the premenstrual temptation time by reducing calorie intake below your usual allowance on three or four 'easy' days at another time of the month.

If this doesn't work, you might just resign yourself to taking a diet holiday for three or four days each month. It is highly unlikely that you will eat enough during that short period to undo all the good work of the rest of the month! But to keep your eating within reasonable bounds the sensible thing is to pre-plan your activity during Big T time so that you are busy, occupied and out of the house as much as possible.

All the solutions arise from recognizing this problem, being aware when it is likely to arise and accepting that determination and willpower alone might not be sufficient to see you through. Pre-plan for Big T time.

'Proper' meals

There's temptation – temptation to eat much more than you really want – in that popular concept of a 'proper meal'. Step inside the home of Mrs A and you will see just what we mean.

Throughout the morning a slice of fruit pie lying in the fridge has been very much on the mind of Mrs A. Her thoughts have kept wandering back to it as she made the beds and tidied the house. But – good for Mrs A – she resisted!

Now, thank goodness, it is lunch time. Now Mrs A can legitimately eat that slice of fruit pie as her dessert. She looks around to see what she can eat as the first course of her meal and decides on some cheese and salad. She eats her way through that and then embarks, at last, on her slice of fruit pie.

All that Mrs A really wanted was that slice of fruit pie!

In order to justify it and eat it in a legitimate way, she ate her way through several hundred calories of cheese.

Most people tend to have a very fixed idea of what constitutes a proper meal. A proper meal, they feel, must always include some high protein food such as meat, cheese or eggs, and it must always include vegetables. Anything which tastes sweet is certainly not a 'proper meal', it can only be eaten as the second course of a meal!

In a society where nutritional deficiencies are rare, and where most people are eating more protein than they need, this too-rigid attitude tempts many people into eating a great deal of unnecessary food.

But won't Mrs A's 'proper meal' protect her against the eating urges of the afternoon? Very probably not. Irrespective of the state of fullness of her stomach, she may well be tempted to snack around 4 o'clock simply because she feels bored, or in response to any of the other appetite triggers listed in this book. At that time the cheese, if not already consumed, could have been used to satisfy a much more compelling desire for food.

If you are trying to control your weight, don't be tempted to eat food you could easily do without, just because it's mealtime.

Reading and eating and eating and reading and . . .

This habit of eating as you are reading can tempt you to

read more (good!) but also to eat more (bad!). Here's the typical situation. You settle down in a comfortable armchair with a good book and a bowl of nuts but, just before the end of the chapter, you run out of nuts. So, you get more nuts to see you through the chapter. The nuts outlast the chapter so you launch into the next chapter to finish up the nuts but, just before the end of that chapter . . .

If you eat while you read, you will be tempted to continue eating for as long as you continue reading, and vice versa. And rarely does the last word of a chapter coincide with the last of the food you have served yourself.

Eating while reading is a bad idea. Turn over a new leaf – don't ever start to eat when you open a book.

Restaurant dessert trolleys

Restaurant desserts are often put on a trolley, on open display, to tempt you to order them – even if you didn't plan to at the start of the meal.

Make some deliberate plans to countcract this deliberate temptation.

There are a variety of ways to prevent the dessert trolley from creeping up on you and tempting you into eating more calories than you intended to eat. Don't let it surprise you. Accept that it's going to be there – it is! So start thinking about how you are going to deal with this temptation before you even step into the restaurant.

If you are familiar with the restaurant, you are probably also familiar with the type of desserts usually on display. You can therefore make a decision in advance – either that you aren't going to have a dessert (you'd rather spend your calories on savoury courses) or that you *are* going to have a dessert (you will cut down calories or cut out a course to allow for it).

It is more difficult if you are going to an unfamiliar restaurant. Here's where the sudden sight of a glorious and unexpected gâteau can rock your self-control at the end of a meal when you know that you've already eaten to your calorie limit in the form of savoury foods: 'Oh well . . . go on . . . I will.'

One woman we know worked out an excellent and much-to-be-recommended method to save herself from dangerous surprises at that vulnerable end-of-meal moment. She makes a point – we suggest you do too – of inspecting the dessert trolley first, whenever she walks into a new restaurant. This is another good advance decision-making time. Is there anything there that is really going to tempt you? If so, by recognizing it before you order the meal you can allow for it by limiting calories in other courses.

In the ideal situation in which you are lunching or dining with another weight-conscious person, you can take the opposite approach of trying to avoid the sight of the dessert trolley. If you both decide in advance that you are not going to eat dessert, you can ask for a table which is well away from the dessert display – and answer the waiter's question, 'Would you like to see the dessert trolley?' with a mutual 'No, thank you'.

Rewards (dangerous)

'If I lose seven pounds in the next three weeks I'll let myself have a great big blow-out in a Chinese restaurant!'

Food-related rewards like this are very dangerous. Quite often, after so much saliva-producing anticipation, the meal does not live up to your expectations. Few things that are too long and too eagerly anticipated ever do quite live up to expectations! So you feel a little disappointed after that 'blow-out'. You also have a sense of having lost ground in your weight-loss programme. You feel that you've wasted a good deal of that effort and that the reward wasn't really worth it anyway!

Food rewards are bad rewards for interim weight loss. They often bring a slimming campaign to a full stop.

If you are yearning for a particular food, whether it is a bar of chocolate or a helping of sweet and sour pork, it is much better to work out how you can include this in your dieting programme, perhaps by 'banking' some calories on easy-to-diet days, than to offer it to yourself in the form of a reward for several weeks' good conduct.

Rewards (unrealistic)

Many people have the tendency to set up a rewards system when they embark on a weight-loss programme. They will reward themselves with something nice every time they shed another three pounds or seven pounds etc. Not a bad idea at all! A rewards system can help to sustain motivation. But it has to be the right kind of rewards system – the wrong one can either prove useless or even tempt you to break your diet.

Often, people promise themselves rewards that are so inconsequential that they don't really care about them. Or they promise themselves, in return for losing a certain amount of weight in a certain amount of time, something they want *so* much that they are going to have it anyway! On *not* achieving their goal, they go ahead and treat themselves to that 'reward' – adding the uncomfortable feeling of disappointment. This puts them very much in the frame of mind to abandon their diet along with their 'contract'!

If you promise yourself rewards, make them realistic, something you really want but not something you are determined to have! The best rewards are those associated with appearance – clothes, make-up, hairdos. These most encourage you to keep on trying to look better and better.

'Room for dessert' syndrome

You have finished the main course of your meal. Your hunger is satisfied. So satisfied that if someone were to urge you to have another helping you would answer: 'No, honestly, I just couldn't eat it . . .'

Then comes the sweet course. Not only do you find that you *can* find room for dessert but often you find it hard to resist the enormous temptation to eat dessert.

There is always a great temptation to have a different taste at the end of a meal. It is the anticipation of another taste sensation, rather than a desire to eat more food, which is persuading you to add a whole load of extra calories to those you have already eaten.

Most people are tempted by a sweet taste at the end of the main meal. Even the drinks – liqueurs – served after a meal tend to be much sweeter than those served at other times. Other people will look for a very sharp, strong taste sensation, like the taste of cheese.

All right – so now you know what you are really after: it's not food, it's a 'taste'! The best solution to this temptation is to work out how you can get this taste at the smallest cost in calories.

Often something very small but very sweet will satisfy the taste craving at a much lower cost in calories than a whole dish of dessert: a chocolate mint cream, perhaps, or a piece of Turkish delight . . . We are very habit-locked into eating certain foods at certain times, but there is no real reason why sweet foods normally reserved for snack-eating should not be used in place of conventional dessert dishes if you find, as you well might, that just a very small unit will satisfy your desire to end a meal with a sweet taste in your mouth.

Another trick worth trying: try stealing just one spoonful of someone else's dessert!

Saving the best for last

Children have a habit of saving the best food on the plate to be eaten last. That cherry on the trifle is carefully set aside to be savoured in that final moment! Grown-ups sometimes forget to discontinue this habit, which means that they are always going to finish all they are served in order to eat their favourite foods.

Reverse this process. Always eat the most desirable foods first in order to counteract this temptation to clear your plate.

Seasonal celebrations

Traditionally, Christmas, Easter and other seasonal celebrations involve the preparation and serving of specially attractive and bountiful food.

Many people inevitably end up still struggling to shed their Christmas-gained pounds at midsummer.

Logically, it is sensible to appreciate that *no one* has ever become overweight because they overate on Christmas Day, Easter Sunday and their birthday. This brings us to the real scenario behind those celebration weight gains . . .

We often begin to prepare for these seasonal celebrations way in advance of the holiday. Urged on by slogans like 'shop early for Christmas', we tend to get caught up in shopping and cooking for the holiday weeks in advance. We feel rather proud of our efficiency in preparing so early.

Food bought or cooked well in advance sits there in the kitchen until we become tempted to eat it. Often we *do* eat it, which leaves us with a problem: now we've got to go out to the shops again to provide more food for the holiday.

Sometimes this cycle will repeat itself two or three times until finally, two days before the festive occasion, we buy or cook the food that will actually be used on that day. In the meantime we have already indulged in two or three calorie-laden 'festive occasions'.

Shops are well aware of this little human failing. By urging us to 'shop early for Christmas' they know they will also encourage us to 'eat early for Christmas' – and end up buying at least twice as much food.

The best solution is to wait until only two or three days before a festive occasion before shopping and cooking. But there are some compromises and alternatives that can be used.

If a great deal of food preparation is necessary, first prepare all the foods which are least tempting to you personally. Wait until the last minute to buy and cook the foods that you have the most difficulty in resisting. Alternatively, if you own a freezer, store the foods there immediately after cooking so that at least you are safe from instant impulse eating.

The next major temptation time arises *after* the seasonal celebration. This is the period when most people, having over-generously stored food for the festivities, continue to wade their way through the calorie-crammed leftovers.

As soon as the celebration is over, make some definite decision about how you are going to use up the leftovers, otherwise you will be tempted to overeat them haphazardly. See the sections of this book on Leftovers for specific advice.

Shopping when hungry

The more hungry you are while shopping, the more tempting and unnecessary food you will buy – and the more you will eat when you get home. And probably continue to eat for the next day or two, as well.

Never shop when you are hungry. Deliberately choose times of day when you know you won't be hungry; straight after lunch, for instance.

Sickbed sympathizers

Since life is crammed with situations which tempt us to eat, it is important to take full advantage of those less frequent situations which tempt us not to eat, such as a helpful cold in the head which dulls appetite, or a useful tummy bug. Golden opportunities, these, for shedding a little weight without any particular effort.

Or they would be, were it not for sickbed sympathizers!

When your appetite is depressed by a minor ailment, your near and dear ones will devote themselves to restoring it. Tirelessly they will cook hot nourishing soup, shop for appetite-tempting delicacies, prepare calorie-crammed drinks and present offerings of chocolates and grapes at your sickbed.

This desire to make you eat stems largely from a health fallacy. People tend to believe that food is necessary to fight the germs and 'keep your strength up'. In the case of overweight adults suffering minor illnesses of short duration, this is not true. Whether you eat or don't eat will make no difference to the duration of a cold. You can safely let your appetite be your guide. The energy your body needs to 'keep its strength up' is safely tucked up in bed in the form of your surplus fat.

Reassure your sickbed sympathizers with these facts.

They may feel comforted if you take vitamin pills, which will cost you nothing in calories!

But another reason for all these little offerings on trays may be your own behaviour. When we are ill most of us tend to regress to childhood behaviour and demand that extra fuss that was the bonus of childhood ailments. Many a fearless captain of industry becomes a petulant oversized baby when he suffers from a cold in the head.

It is interesting to note that we also tend to revert to childhood food when we aren't feeling well. The captain of industry might well be found dunking his bread into his soft-boiled egg, or spooning up a bowl of rice pudding — possibly having requested it to be served with a dollop of jam!

Faced with our petulant demands for extra fuss our sickbed sympathizers, poor souls, often find it difficult to think of what they *can* do for us — apart from preparing food. This leaves us with the options of either suffering more food silently or diverting their efforts to providing comforts unrelated to food such as books and magazines.

When you aren't feeling well, try to separate the fuss that you need from the food that you can quite easily do without.

Sleeplessness

You are lying in bed, unable to get to sleep. The person lying next to you is contentedly dreaming or snoring. Maybe you are worried about something, maybe you just don't need the sleep, maybe you have gone to bed too early.

After the first fifteen minutes of tossing and turning you start to wonder what you can do to make yourself sleepy. Often the first thing that comes to mind is eating. If you are dieting, a certain food down there in the kitchen is likely to be very much on your mind.

There's a good chance that you went to bed early in order to avoid eating it!

What can you do?

There are several ways to handle this situation. One way is to get up and go and do something else like taking a hot bath which can be very relaxing. Or at least switch on the light and read for a while. If you lie there long enough just thinking about the food, you are going to go and get it.,

If you are really craving for a particular food, try to work out how you can include some of that food in tomorrow's calorie allowance. If you know that you can have a tempting food tomorrow, its importance today often diminishes.

If neither of these tactics works, our advice to you is to go and have a small portion of that particular food. Deliberately cut off a small portion, sit down with it downstairs and eat it slowly. Don't take it back upstairs. Eating in bed is a poor sport. Nobody likes crumbs in bed! For the slimmer it is a particularly poor sport because if you get into the habit of eating in bed the bedroom begins to acquire a subconscious association with food. Pretty soon you can even find yourself acquiring the habit of walking upstairs to bed each night with a plate of food in your hand.

The worst thing to do about night-time cravings is to try to stave off the craving for a particular food by the use of another food. If you crave a piece of chocolate cake which is sitting in the kitchen and go down to the kitchen to eat a piece of fruit or some celery or ryecrisps, you are brought into close proximity with the craved food, which is likely to intensify the craving.

Usually what happens is something like this: you go downstairs and help yourself to an apple and eat the apple. You go back upstairs hoping that you will now get off to sleep and stop thinking of that chocolate cake. You do not get off to sleep. You do not stop thinking of that chocolate cake. Maybe something a little sweeter would help. You go downstairs again and help yourself to a small bowl of cereal. You eat the cereal and return to bed hoping that this will take care of the problem. Generally it doesn't. That wretched chocolate cake is *still* on your mind.

You give up, you get up, you go downstairs and help yourself to a large lump of chocolate cake – and then, more likely than not, another lump. What the hell. What's the use!

You have now eaten an apple, a bowl of breakfast cereal and a lump of chocolate cake in addition to your calorie allowance, so there seems little point in putting on the brakes at this stage . . .

That's why it's better to eat a little, in a controlled way, than to try these usually doomed diversionary tactics.

Superhuman willpower

Many humans ruin their weight-loss prospects by succumbing to the temptation to be superhuman.

Typical situation: you accept an invitation to a social occasion at which you know you will be watching everyone else doing a vast amount of eating and drinking. You resolve hardly to eat a thing yourself. And to drink nothing but low-calorie tonics.

Maybe you even succeed.

The trouble is, the situation often doesn't end there. Very often you go home feeling very deprived. Very often people in this state of mind will eventually succumb to a snack when they get home. On eating a snack after refusing all that lovely food you then tend to feel rather annoyed with yourself. On feeling annoyed with yourself you then easily get into the kind of mood that can turn a snack into a binge. Very often people who deprive themselves too strictly on social occasions go home and end up eating many more calories in private than they would had they eaten in company with everyone else.

There are a variety of much better ways in which to deal with a temptation-packed social occasion. You could decide to give it a miss altogether. Or you could save calories during the day or during several previous days in order to allow yourself to indulge in moderation. The worst way to deal with a highly tempting social occasion is to use it to put your willpower to a superhuman test.

Supermarkets

When you step into a supermarket you are stepping into a minefield of temptation. Proceed with the utmost caution. Take every step with care – even avoid stepping into some danger zones at all.

In recent years, on both sides of the Atlantic, supermarket tycoons have had to face a growing problem. The problem is that the population has stopped growing – in numbers, that is!

In order to increase the sales, the logical object of every efficient food retailer is now to persuade each member of the population to cram down *more* food during every twenty-four-hour period.

Make no mistake about it, they're out to get you! And they have carefully worked-out ways of sabotaging your food control. Awareness is the main countermeasure to use against these slimming saboteurs.

Look what they're up to! It's no accident that those packets of crisps and crunchy between-meal nibbles are piled in wire containers which jut out in the aisle, all set for a collision with your shopping cart. They almost drop right into your cart, don't they? Sometimes they actually *do*! It's all intentional. A carefully worked-out ploy to attract you to an extra 'buy'.

Equally intentional is the fact that tempting savoury nibbles are nearly always offered in transparent packaging. Technological testing suggests that they could be stored for longer periods in opaque containers. But sales research shows that if you actually *see* food, you are much more likely to buy it and eat it. Sight is an important appetite trigger.

If you want to know which are the supermarket's most highly profitable lines, they can usually be spotted in the areas you are destined to pass most frequently as you wander around – often the food display that runs right along the far end and comes in view every time you reach the end of an aisle.

The supermarket tycoon knows that the more often you see a certain food, the more likely you are to buy it. Take combat countermeasures in this struggle by working out how you can avoid constant glimpses of your biggest temptations.

Never wander around a supermarket haphazardly. Plan your moves. Consider the location of your greatest temptation and ask yourself whether you really need to go along that aisle at all.

It is no accident that child-tempting foods are displayed at junior eye level. Resist the temptation of telling yourself: 'Well, I'll buy it for the children but I won't eat any myself!' Children's foods are often very tempting to adults.

It's also no accident that calorie-crammed sweets and confectioneries are displayed right by the check-out counter, ready and waiting to provide the knock-out punch if you have so far resisted all visual temptations. Here they have you trapped – a prisoner – eye to eye with a chocolate-coated munchy bar for as long as it takes to stand in the check-out line and pay for your food.

A shopping list, a firm resolve to buy nothing you haven't 'listed', and a full awareness of all the traps deliberately set to tempt you to buy more and eat more are your best weapons in the supermarket sabotage game.

Sweetening coffee

This is a singular temptation in that for many people it simply doesn't exist at all.

Many people are *always* tempted to add extra calories by sugaring coffee. Just as many more are *never* tempted. Very few people are 'sometimes' tempted!

Indeed, people who are not in the habit of sweetening their coffee are usually repelled by the idea of drinking it sweet.

It is usually possible to cross the great divide, we find, in a period of about three weeks' abstinence. Or a slightly longer period if you opt for the easier method of reducing sweetness little by little.

Resolute action is worthwhile for such permanent rewards.

Once this habit is cured it is usually cured for the rest of your life, which leaves you with a mere ninety-nine temptations to tackle in the future!

Television advertisements

TV food advertisements are deliberately calculated to urge you to eat more food. Very often they are all too effective. And this isn't the least bit surprising!

Here's a real David and Goliath contest if ever there was one. It features you, often at the time of the day when you are least armed against temptation, in contest with all the subtle skills of the mighty advertising industry.

One of the most honest advertisements we recall (for a

brand of cigars, if memory serves us right) featured a cheerful chap who waved his cigar at the screen with the comment: 'We're going to get you – sooner or later we're going to get you!'

And that's the trouble. Sooner or later they *are* likely to get you, in some vulnerable moment, if you aren't very careful. So what can you do?

We'll rule out not watching TV as even more sacrificial than not eating food, for most people. Of course, you can get up and go out of the room every time the advertisements start, which would involve you in a good deal of beneficial physical activity. But that is going to be a pretty tiresome chore, and the danger is that your feet might well be tempted to head towards the kitchen. Keeping a magazine handy is probably the only semi-practical 'don't watch them' approach to the problem.

Assuming that most people will be watching those advertisements, the best countermeasure, we find, lies in developing an awareness of *how* they are trying to get you! It's the subtle, almost subliminal message that usually slips through and proves most tempting. And by developing an interest in the technique of advertising itself you at least part-divert your attention from the food that is being advertised.

Become a television advertising critic. Get out your big cigar (well, mentally, at least) and sit and deliver judgment on the skills or otherwise of the advertising agency that is presenting its efforts for your inspection.

This way you might well find yourself thinking: 'Now *that* was a good advertisement!' rather than '*That* was a delicious, meaty, flavour-packed beefburger!'

It is endlessly intriguing to discover the many ways in which the advertising agencies attempt to appeal to us. Sometimes they aim for our sense of humour to give us a warm, friendly fellow-feeling towards the food being advertised. Often they aim at maternal or wifely instincts, giving a subtle impression that not to serve this particular breakfast cereal or supper is to deprive the family.

Many advertisements even aim at our patriotism, leaving a marked impression that not to eat this particular food is decidely un-British!

A very large percentage of advertisements aim at our natural desire for good looks, good health and vitality. Often, because the food actually being advertised has little to do with any of these assets, the suggestion is made in an indirect way. The lovely girl drinking that fizzy drink or eating that chocolate bar is leaping about in such a lithe and energetic way that the impression is created that by drinking or eating the same thing we too will be galvanized into such life and loveliness!

Perhaps the most effective antidote of all lies in being aware that if you are overweight, succumbing to the message of any food advertisement is almost certain to have precisely the opposite effect to the one being suggested. Energy is just another word for calories – excess energy is stored as surplus fat, and that makes us less energetic. Better looks and health can rarely be achieved by eating more of any particular food. They can often be achieved by eating less. Excess weight is no laughing matter – as you know yourself. And, come to think of it, government health advisers are deeply concerned about the hazards caused by widespread obesity. It is even a little un-British to eat more!

TGIF!

Yes, indeed, Thank God it's Friday! Friday signals the start of the weekend – a mini festival during which we reward ourselves for all the efforts and disciplines of the week.

Weekend often includes that big family Sunday lunch, the Saturday night dinner party, or the big leisurely cooked breakfast. Nearly all festivals and rewards tend to include food!

Be aware that, as far as eating patterns are concerned, Saturdays and Sundays are quite different from the other five days of the week – and often considerably more tempting.

We once asked a hundred women, who had all succeeded in achieving that elusive goal of shedding *all* their surplus weight, to list the greatest temptation they had had to overcome during their dieting programme. Weekends stood out as the major temptation for the majority!

But these were successful dieters, so presumably they had kept strictly to their diets each weekend by gritting their teeth? Not so! Most, we discovered, had adapted their diets to allow for some degree of weekend indulgence and reward – a few alcoholic drinks in some cases, or a few cakes or snacks, or a generous helping of that big Sunday lunch.

'I can be very strict all week, as long as I can look forward to letting up a bit at the weekend,' was a typical comment.

For most people, that is the best way to cope with the eating temptations of the weekend. If Saturdays and Sundays are the days on which you find it specially difficult to control your eating, accept that fact. Try to cut down calories a little more during the easier weekdays in order to allow yourself planned rather than accidental weekend indulgences.

The last piece

The last piece of food, lying in an almost empty packet or

tin, can present you with the temptation to eat in order to be tidy.

You are tidying out the kitchen or a cupboard, you would like to throw that box away; in order to do so, you pop that last piece of food into your mouth . . .

Tidiness can tempt you to eat unless you learn to throw away that last piece – or become a little less tidy!

Thin friends

A thin friend may try to tempt you to stop dieting! Probably not at first – particularly if you are quite heavily overweight. In the initial stages your slim friend might be quite encouraging. After all, she's experienced your dieting attempts before. Probably she is fairly confident that this attempt will fail too, or at least that you will give up when you have lost just some of your surplus weight.

Her sabotage tactics – 'I really think you've lost enough!' – are more likely to start midway through your slimming campaign when it starts to become apparent that you have now become considerably less fat and are well on your way to becoming as thin as she is.

Part of the basis of some friendships between an overweight woman and a slim woman is the factor that the overweight woman acts as a 'foil'. The slim woman feels more slim and attractive by comparison. This is something that your thin friend has come to accept and to some degree enjoy.

Overweight women tend to be non-competitive in the sexual areas. Even if you are both happily married, your friend may enjoy the fact that she is the one who always attracts the compliments from men, and you don't try to compete.

Overweight women also have a tendency to be non-assertive. If you are overweight and she is thin, it is probable that you will be the one who tends to fit in with her plans.

You will see that by becoming slim you will tend to make quite a lot of changes in this relationship. Again, it is natural for your slim friend to resist these changes. And this friendship may possibly dissolve when you become thin, more sexually attractive, more sure of yourself and more assertive. Don't fear changes like this; there are very many people in the world with whom you can form friendships, and becoming slim will often lead you to form friendships more easily.

Be aware that thin friends might start to discourage you from dieting when you are in sight of your goal, so that those 'you've lost enough' comments won't put dangerous doubts in your mind.

Thirst

The day is hot, the task is energetic – and suddenly you find yourself suffering from an enormous thirst. At this moment a favourite soft drink, or maybe the prospect of a beer, becomes enormously tempting. You open a can, pour it down, open another . . . you carry on drinking until the thirst is quenched. By this time you can have poured down an awful lot of calories. Here's a policy that will save you from many of them in the future.

Make a habit of quenching thirst before you drink your favourite calorie-supplying drinks. Satisfy your need for liquid with iced water, iced tea or another low-calorie drink. Then you can safely allow yourself that favourite drink without being tempted to drink large quantities.

In fact we hardly really notice the taste of that first drink, gulped down quickly in response to thirst. It is only when thirst is quenched that we become fully aware of taste. Quench your thirst before you consume your calories.

Transitional eating

Those chores of the day are finished at last. Time to relax! If this situation always starts you heading for the kitchen, you are responding to a temptation called 'transitional eating'.

There is a common urge to emphasize the transition from one part of the day to another by turning to food. Food is used to put the punctuation marks into the day – to bring one period to an end with a firm full stop. Be aware of this, try to achieve the same satisfying sense of transition by other means.

Home from work? Try changing out of those formal clothes and maybe taking a stroll. The children in bed at last? A relaxing soak in a mid-evening bath can act as an excellent unwinder. Work out ways of putting transitional breaks into the day without using food for this purpose.

Unexpected pieces of time

Life is never one hundred per cent predictable. It is frequently punctuated with unexpected pieces of time. Maybe you are waiting at a station and hear that your train is going to be delayed. Maybe you are at home and a friend who was going to visit phones to say she can't make it. Perhaps you have simply finished your household tasks more quickly than you had expected. Or your husband phones to say he will be late home for dinner . . .

All these situations, and many, many more, present you with an unexpected piece of time; and the problem of how to fill it; and a *great* temptation to eat, because an almost automatic reaction is to make yourself a cup of coffee and assuage boredom (the most dangerous mood for slimmers) with a snack.

Be aware that unexpected pieces of time crop up frequently in your life, most frequently in your home. Prepare for them.

A helpful countermeasure is to have some easily picked-up hobby or project available around the house. Some knitting or embroidery, perhaps, that you can turn to with a certain amount of pleasure to fill that odd half hour.

A useful investment is a few new paperback books – not the kind you feel you 'ought' to read but the kind you really want to read. If you are in the middle of an absorbing book, you'll welcome the unexpected opportunity to pick it up again. Magazines can be even better, if you resist the temptation to read them when they arrive and save them to relish with unexpected pleasure during that unexpected piece of time.

An alternative is to have a list of household tasks-to-be-accomplished to turn to in a deliberate way – so that you have essentially laid a plan, in advance, for unexpected time. We know of one slimmer who emptied her biscuit jar and filled it with pieces of paper, each listing a household task and assessing the approximate time of the task. In her case it worked, largely because she'd recognized unexpected pieces of time as an eating temptation, and prepared for them.

Expect unexpected pieces of time.

Unpacking shopping

On returning from a shopping expedition the average housewife proceeds to unload all the food from her bags and pile it on to the kitchen table.

She's feeling a little tired. So probably she sits down for a minute or two, and . . .

Found yourself nibbling something or other in

moments like this?

It's hardly surprising. You're tired, and tiredness lessens self-control. And you are sitting right in front of a whole load of temptation. Unpacking shopping in this way provides a great eating temptation.

To avoid it, take a little break when you arrive home from the shops. Make yourself a cup of coffee, glance through the newspaper for a few minutes to relax and unwind. *Then* start to unpack your shopping. Take your purchases out of the bag, one at a time, and as you unwrap each food, put it away in its appropriate cupboard or container before unloading the next one. And make sure that anything particularly tempting is put in a container that covers it up – so that it won't keep asking you to eat it every time you open a cupboard door.

Untypical days

This is not a typical day. You are more (less!) busy than usual. You are going out (or staying in). The family will be in (out) all day. You are more worried (carefree) than usual . . . the weather is exceptionally good (bad) . . . everything (nothing) is happening . . . you've had bad (good) news . . .

Save yourself from an everyday temptation to eat more than you had planned by accepting one simple fact of life. There is no such thing as a typical day.

Variety

Scientists, attempting to fatten up rats, have found that the best method is to offer them a more varied diet. Given a selection of foods rather than one staple food, the rats will eat more and gain weight. The same has been found true of other animals in fattening-up experiments.

It is certainly true of human beings! The diet of the Western world is very varied, which is good for nutritional requirements but bad for weight. The fact that most of our meals consist of a variety of different foods, and often several different courses, is one of the major factors which tempts us to eat more than we need to satisfy our hunger.

It is almost as if we have to reach the right degree of satiety with each food. Having satisfied our appetite for that food, and switched to one of different taste and texture, we start almost back at square one in seeking satiety again. After consuming a bowl of soup we find that we have had sufficient and lack any further desire to eat more soup. But this has little effect in lowering our appetites when we embark on the meat and vegetable course. Variety in taste and texture of food is certainly one of the greatest appetite stimulants.

At least one medical expert we know, experimenting in the field of obesity, is beginning to wonder whether the common practice of making diets as varied as possible is such a good thing after all. Certainly every obesity expert knows that if the food choice of any overweight person is restricted to just one or two foods, this will result in an inevitable reduction of calorie intake – even if those two foods are doughnuts and cream cakes! Without variety, our appetites severely diminish.

The temptation of our varied Western diet is a tough one to tackle, and a certain amount of variety is necessary to ensure that all nutritional requirements are met. But if you are aware that the more variety you offer yourself the more you will want to eat at any single sitting, there are sometimes ways in which you can decrease this temptation.

Generally a two-course meal is safer than a three-course

meal, and a single-course meal is better still. Housewives who make a habit of serving their families with a three-course dinner every evening are setting themselves up for a very strong temptation.

At breakfast time, a multi-course meal is a particularly bad idea. By eating cereal, cooked food, then toast, it is easy to down a thousand calories, which is about half the average woman's calorie requirement for a day. We very much doubt that most people would approach this calorie intake in a single course of cereal or a cooked dish or toast, however generously they ate.

Waiters

Waiters are employed to help you, to serve you – and also to tempt you to eat more food!

In an *à la carte* restaurant, the more courses you eat, the more you pay. Also, the more you tip, because your tip is usually based on a percentage of the bill. The waiter knows that, so he has a vested interest in encouraging you to eat more. Hence the speed with which the dessert trolley tends to appear at the table, unless you swiftly pre-empt this move with a firm: 'No dessert – just coffee, please.'

Good waiters aim to please, and know that what pleases most customers is the satisfaction of getting a large quantity of food for their money. Hence, in an inclusive menu they are quick to point out that the soup and bread roll are included as part of the meal – should you decide to skip this course. Anticipate these comments in making the wise decision that you don't *have* to eat everything you pay for.

And don't feel (as some people do!) that you *have* to finish your meal for fear of upsetting that nice, helpful waiter who recommended it. Simply reply, 'It was very good – but just a little more than I could eat,' if he asks if there was anything wrong with it.

Waiters sometimes should be asked to wait. In many restaurants another part of their job is to encourage you to get through your meal at maximum speed in order to free the table for other customers. The next course appears on the table the moment the plates are cleared. Don't hesitate to tell the waiter: 'We'd like to take ten minutes before the next course.' A meal eaten at a more leisurely pace gives more pleasure and satisfies the appetite for longer.

Waiters are there to provide personal service but, often, overweight people with their fear of 'drawing attention to themselves' are too hesitant to make special requests, perhaps for a coffee to be served before a meal, or for the salad to be served without its usual dressing, which could help them to control their calorie intake. That is why, as part of behavioural weight-control programmes, patients are asked to practise by making some special request even if it is just for another glass of water, every time they eat a restaurant meal.

Waiters can be bad for your weight if you let them set the pace and dictate the quantity – helpful if you learn and practise the gently assertive art of customer control.

Waiting . . .

Waiting is boring, and boredom is the foremost appetite-stimulating mood. Waiting is tiring, unless there is somewhere to sit – and often the only place to sit is in a café or restaurant. Waiting presents you with an unexpected piece of time, and the automatic urge to fill it with food. Waiting is often a slightly anxious time (Will the plane arrive? Have I remembered the right meeting place?), and many people eat in response to anxiety.

An awful lot of people spend an awful lot of time waiting. Among them is Audrey Eyton, one of the authors of this book.

In 1978, on Washington Station, Audrey Eyton experienced a unique happening in her own lifetime (an all-time personal 'best') by running along a platform and catching a train with less than half a second to spare.

A clear case of cutting it almost too fine?

Not at all. She had arrived so early for her scheduled train that it suddenly became apparent that she could catch a train leaving one and a half hours earlier.

She is far from being the only compulsively early person in this world.

Probably there are a few people who have a happy knack of always arriving just on time. But, largely, the world is divided into two types of people, those who always arrive early and those who always arrive late.

Psychological studies have shown that the always-late person is strongly compulsive in this habit. Late people seem to need the excitement and stimulation of 'cutting it fine'. Often they subconsciously create delaying situations which will necessitate a last-minute departure.

A psychiatrist friend of ours, well aware of this fact, once decided to get an always-late colleague to his party on time. So he used the only practical technique, which was to pull the party-starting time forward by two hours when he issued the invitation. Unfortunately this turned out to be the one time in his life when the guest arrived precisely on time, and his host had to greet him in his underwear. But such departures from habit are very rare!

The always-early person is just as compulsive as the always-late. Without that 'just in case anything goes wrong' time built in, he finds any journey filled with too many anxieties. Hence he spends a large part of his life in a situation that is packed with eating temptations – waiting!

One solution to this problem could be to work consciously at getting there just on time, or even to be wildly risky and discover that the world doesn't end when you deliberately get there even a few minutes late. This solution is unlikely to work. Inevitably, the day on which you try your experiment will be the day on which you do become ensnarled in a two–hour traffic jam, miss the friend you were meeting and go home swearing: 'Never again!'

We once read this advice in a splendid little book called *How to make yourself thoroughly miserable*: 'Set off to the airport fifteen minutes late and with your petrol tank indicator hovering on "empty".' For the compulsively early person this is certainly guaranteed to induce a nervous breakdown.

The most realistic solution to the waiting–eating problem lies in simply accepting that you will arrive early. Accept those extra pieces of time and consider how you will fill them. Don't let them take you by surprise for the five thousandth time.

Various time-filling solutions may present themselves to you, from always going to meetings equipped with a good book, or even taking your knitting along. But, quite possibly, eating will still turn out to be the most convenient and satisfactory way to fill most periods of waiting time. In which case, plan to eat. But plan to eat as part of your usual daily food quota, rather than in the form of extra snacks. Journeys usually follow meals. In most situations you set off after breakfast, lunch or dinner. Simply delay breakfast, lunch or dinner to be eaten in any handy restaurant or cafeteria near your meeting place, thus comfortably filling your waiting time without guilt, by eating non–illicit food.

'You ought to eat something!'

Sooner or later, as you launch off on your weight-loss campaign, you will be tempted to eat because someone warns you, with a worried look, that 'you really ought to eat something!'

You are setting off on a journey: 'You ought to eat something first,' advises your nearest and dearest. You are about to go out on a chilly day: 'You ought to eat something on a day like this!' You have decided to skip lunch on a particularly busy day, when your best friend warns with a note of deep concern: 'But don't you think you ought to have at least a little something!'

Then, quite often, you *do* eat something. Something that you didn't really need. Because deep down in most people lurks a hidden fear that something quite diabolical will happen if they go for more than a few hours without eating something.

Consider the facts to offset this temptation. Even the normal-weight person, carrying no surplus fat, can survive without food for nearly a month, the overweight person for much longer. Health-giving nutrients do not have to be fed in at regular intervals throughout the day, vitamins and minerals only need to be adequately consumed over periods of several days, even weeks. Long gaps between meals are not generally harmful to the health of the normal person. If you are overweight, there is nothing that food can do to offset cold or fatigue that your own body fat can't do just as adequately! And that gives you the bonus of weight loss!

So what is the worst that can happen if you *don't* eat something? In extreme cases some people feel faint after lengthy periods without food. But, assuming that you aren't rowing across the Atlantic on a raft, you are unlikely ever to be in a situation where food cannot be obtained within minutes should this problem arise in this food-crammed Western world. Some people may experience hunger pangs, but those usually quickly fade of their own accord even without the aid of food. And those are the only food-gap hazards we can think of.

Don't eat something because someone feels that you

ought to. If *you* don't feel the need, and are overweight, don't eat.

You

You – not fate – will determine your own weight. And people who turn to alibis or blame circumstances around them for weight problems tempt themselves to fail in food control.

Temptations abound, that's true. You have just read a whole bookful of them, which apply to other people as well as to you. Now that you are more aware, better equipped to deal with them, you won't beat the lot (perfectionism is a dangerous policy) but the lot won't beat you! You make a big step forward towards a permanently slim figure each time you learn to eliminate or tackle a single food temptation. You can achieve your goal while still succumbing to quite a few. So aim at steady progress.

Now, over to you . . .

Brian Inglis

NATURAL MEDICINE

There are few certainties in medicine – fewer now than perhaps at any time – and yet what Arthur Koestler has termed 'the narrow-minded orthodoxy of the medical profession' still predominates. The establishment dismisses other forms of medical practice as being 'fringe', 'alternative', 'unorthodox' and 'paramedical', even though its own approach has often been found to be sadly and cruelly misguided.

But nature cure, herbalism, homeopathy, osteopathy, chiropractics, acupuncture, radiesthesia and healing are not things peddled by quacks for cranks. As Brian Inglis shows, nature has its own healing force (a power which has been used by man from the earliest times to the present day), and this should be assisted, not supplanted, by orthodox medicine to form an integral part of every nation's health service.

This investigation into the history and practice of natural medicine, with its clear and useful explanations and invaluable list of organizations involved, will be of great interest both to the medical profession and to the growing numbers of ordinary people concerned with their health and selfcare. At a time when the public, disillusioned with drugs, is showing an ever-increasing preference for alternative medicine, its importance cannot be exaggerated.

'An extraordinarily interesting book' – the *Tablet*

'. . . a brief, sensible history of the theories and practices that orthodox medicine loves to hate' – Francis Huxley, *Guardian*

Fontana Paperbacks: Non-fiction

Fontana is a leading paperback publisher of non-fiction, both popular and academic. Below are some recent titles.

☐ AN AUTOBIOGRAPHY   Peter Alliss £1·95
☐ BOB HOPE: PORTRAIT OF A SUPERSTAR   Charles Thompson £1·75
☐ SUBJECT WOMEN   Ann Oakley £2·75
☐ HOW TO GET RID OF THE BOMB   Gavin Scott £1·95
☐ POLICEMAN'S PATCH   Harry Cole £1·50
☐ A YEAR IN THE DRINK   Martin Green £1·75
☐ SCOTLAND   introduction by Lord Home £4·95
☐ THE NO-DIET BOOK   Michael Spira £1·50
☐ SIR JAMES GOLDSMITH   Geoffrey Wansell £1·95
☐ THE CINDERELLA COMPLEX   Colette Dowling £1·75
☐ DIANA, THE PRINCESS OF WALES   Hugh Montgomery-Massingberd £1·95
☐ SONIA ALLISON'S FOOD PROCESSOR COOKBOOK   £1·95
☐ THE ENTERTAINING COOKBOOK   Evelyn Rose £3·95
☐ WAR AND SOCIETY IN REVOLUTIONARY EUROPE 1770–1870   Geoffrey Best £2·95
☐ EUROPEAN EMPIRES FROM CONQUEST TO COLLAPSE 1815–1960   Victor Kiernan £2·95
☐ DARWIN   Wilma George £1·75
☐ THIS IS WINDSURFING   Reinhart Winkler £5·95
☐ CHAMPION'S STORY   Bob Champion & Jonathan Powell £1·50

You can buy Fontana paperbacks at your local bookshop or newsagent. Or you can order them from Fontana Paperbacks, Cash Sales Department, Box 29, Douglas, Isle of Man. Please send a cheque, postal or money order (not currency) worth the purchase price plus 10p per book (or plus 12p per book if outside the UK).

NAME (Block letters) _____

ADDRESS _____

_____

_____